With Shaking Hands

Studies in Medical Anthropology

Edited by Mac Marshall

With Shaking Hands

Aging with Parkinson's Disease in America's Heartland

SAMANTHA SOLIMEO

RUTGERS UNIVERSITY PRESS

NEW BRUNSWICK, NEW JERSEY, AND LONDON

LIBRARY OF CONGRESS CATALOGING-IN-PUBLICATION DATA

Solimeo, Samantha, 1974–

    With shaking hands : aging with Parkinson's disease in America's heartland /
Samantha Solimeo.
      p. cm.—(Studies in medical anthropology)
    Includes bibliographical references and index.
    ISBN 978-0-8135-4543-1 (hardcover : alk. paper)
    ISBN 978-0-8135-4544-8 (pbk : alk. paper)
    I. Parkinson's disease—Middle West. 2. Medical anthropology. I. Title. II. Series.
[DNLM: I. Parkinson Disease—psychology—United States—Personal Narratives.
2. Aged—United States. 3. Aging—psychology—United States—Personal
Narratives. 4. Antiparkinson Agents—United States—Personal Narratives.
5. Caregivers—psychology—United States—Personal Narratives. 6. Health
Services for the Aged—United States—Personal Narratives. WL 359 S686w 2009
RC382.S648 2009
362.196833—dc22   2008035435

A British Cataloging-in-Publication record for this book is available
from the British Library.

Copyright © 2009 by Samantha Solimeo

Visit our Web site: http://rutgerspress.rutgers.edu

Manufactured in the United States of America

For my grandparents,
William and Doris Roverano, Charles and Lucy Solimeo,
and Bob and Betty Hillman

CONTENTS

ACKNOWLEDGMENTS

Many people have contributed to this book's success. First, I extend my gratitude to the men and women who welcomed this "young lady from back East" into their homes and lives. I hope that in sharing your stories with dignity I have found a small justice in the face of this challenging condition. Special thanks go to the PD support group facilitators who assisted with recruiting and ongoing research support, particularly John McConeghey, Don Schneider, Wilma Schimmel, and Dot Christiansen.

The University of Iowa provided instrumental and intellectual support during the formative stages of the project. Margery Wolf, Carolyn Hough, and Sarah Ono helped me to understand that feminist anthropology need not be synonymous with studying women and they inspired me to think more deeply about feminist epistemology, methodology, and ethics. Michael Chibnik provided helpful grant-writing advice. Erica Prussing, Maureen McCue, and Toni Tripp-Reimer pushed me to both narrow my focus and develop my independence as a "gero" and medical anthropologist.

Two colleagues in the Association for Anthropology and Gerontology provided critical evaluation of this research at different stages in its development. Annette Leibing and Judith Barker generously provided editorial, methodological, and theoretical feedback that has improved the manuscript in many ways.

The Duke University Center for the Study of Aging and Human Development fostered a critical and stimulating environment for manuscript development. Deborah T. Gold has been of particular support. Beginning in her role as a postdoctoral mentor and continuing today, she has been a tireless advocate and supporter of this research.

Financial support for the research was provided in part by: Parkinson's Disease Foundation Summer Fellowship in Investigative Research; National Science Foundation, Dissertation Research Grant; Department of Health and Human Services, Agency for Healthcare Research and Quality, Dissertation Research Grant; University of Iowa Department of Anthropology, University of Iowa Student Government, Summer Research Grant, and University of Iowa Graduate College, Graduate Incentive Fellowship; and National Institutes of Health, National Institute on Aging Research Training Grant (T32 AG000029).

I wish to acknowledge the support of those colleagues and family closest to the work. Thanks go to Ernie, Sofia, and Aster Cox for their patience with me during this lengthy process. Thanks also to my family for your enthusiasm and encouragement, even in those moments when you weren't sure what it was I was up to. Finally, I am pleased to have this space to publicly thank Mac Marshall. Dr. Marshall has been a colleague for more than ten years. His passion for anthropology and his kind regard for the people behind the words, mine and theirs, have taught me volumes about personhood and quality of life.

ABBREVIATIONS

AD	Alzheimer's disease
CAM	Complementary and alternative medicine
COMT	Catechol-o-methyltransferase inhibitors
COPD	Chronic obstructive pulmonary disease
DA	Dopamine agonist
DBS	Deep brain stimulation
EM	Explanatory model
MAO-B	Monoamine oxidase inhibitors
MS	Multiple sclerosis
PD	Parkinson's disease

With Shaking Hands

1

Introduction

Becoming Old, Becoming Sick

Introduction: Reevaluating What Being Old Is

Leroy and Kathryn live in a modest two-story home on the edge of one of Iowa's few urban centers. They bought their home about forty years ago, shortly after they were married, when Leroy started work as a primary school teacher. Together, Leroy and Kathryn raised a small family and maintained active social lives in their faith and arts communities. Leroy was almost seventy years old when I first met him, and had had Parkinson's disease (PD) for about six years. He was diagnosed just a few years after he retired, and his case had progressed from its simple presentation of fatigue and postural changes to a complex and disabling disorder. Despite his formidable and unpredictable impairments, Leroy maintains an optimistic and lighthearted outlook. As long as he is able to create art, read, attend the occasional play, and spend time with his wife, life with PD is for him a blessing.

Leroy's first signs of PD appeared over a period of months, but because the symptoms emerged while he was undergoing treatment for vertigo, it was quite a while before he and his wife put the pieces together to realize that something was amiss. "Well, thinking back, you can kind of tell something was going wrong," he says. "My first symptom, as far as the PD, was my posture. I had more difficulty standing straight; I was more slumped over. When I would write some-thing, . . . I would start taking notes with a normal hand and by the time I got to the end they were so cramped you couldn't read it. So this was the way it went, you know. I had so much saliva in my mouth, it would actually drool out. And this is because you don't swallow as often as you should. And I was just con-stantly wore out, fatigued." He stopped for a moment to take another dose of carbidopa-levodopa.

When Leroy's symptoms first appeared, he didn't think that anything seri-ous was afoot. "I just thought . . . I was retired and maybe I was just . . . it was something that I didn't expect. When it was finally diagnosed by the neurologist, I really didn't know what PD was. And he gave me a book to read. And I started finding out as much about it as I could." Leroy's was one of the few physicians whom study participants I interviewed described as compassionate and willing to take the time to address his patients' concerns. While Leroy and his wife didn't sink into a depression or actively deny the unwelcome news, a radio show made them realize the gravity of his prognosis. As Kathryn said, "They had interviewed Moe Udall. Well, they didn't interview him, they interviewed his wife. And this wasn't too long after Leroy was diagnosed with it. And he [Udall] was already in the hospital, not able to move. And that was kind of a shocker. That was a downer night for me, anyway."

As surprised as Leroy was to have developed a disorder that he had never heard of, he was more taken aback that this should happen to a healthy person.

> Because I had never been sick. When I left teaching, I had hundreds of sick days built up. . . . I used to run. I jogged in the summer, two to five miles every day. So the illness wasn't something I planned on. [laughs] And I don't know about PD. The doctors have often said that PD patients were in perfectly good health except that they had this one thing wrong with them—and it was an incurable disease! I think that's fairly common with others; they'd had good health up until the point they got it. And the disease is kind of unpredictable in that sense. It is kind of difficult to think of yourself as being ill, to think that I can't go out and do work in the yard or I have a restriction on my driver's license. It's hard to accept it. I don't dwell on it. I don't brood over it. Kathryn does most of the driving now. I see her out mowing the yard and I should be out doing that myself. It's hard to get used to, in that sense.

Leroy and I discussed how he felt when the medicines were at their peak efficacy. Did he feel disabled? Normal? His response reveals the complexity of embodiment in PD. In the moments when persons with PD feel fully themselves, there always lingers the knowledge that this normalcy is fleeting. It changes with each moment, each medication dose, each month, each year. Aging, medication side effects, and disease progression conspire to position PD sufferers on unpredictable terrain. As Leroy related, "When they are all working just exactly the way they're supposed to, I don't feel like I'm really that bad off. I mean, it's close to being normal, whatever being normal at sixty-eight is, because I'm not used to being sixty-eight. But I have thought about that. I drive out to the mall and go out and get things and walk around and I feel that I must be almost normal. So when they are working, they still give me a close to normal existence. But you have to constantly keep in mind, 'Maybe I've got an hour or two and then I'm going to get cramps in my feet and fall here on my face.' But I can still get the medicine to work— it's all right."

I asked Leroy to describe a typical day for him. His story elucidates the tragedy of the medication window, the window of time when medications restore normal function, more clearly than those of any of the PD sufferers that I spoke with. Every morning Leroy is wakened by cramps and aches in his feet and lower limbs. He gets out of bed, uses the bathroom, takes his first round of medicines, and gets back into bed until they take effect. Thirty minutes later he is able to get up again, dress, and have breakfast. "If I didn't take the medicine, I'd be in the hospital. I couldn't make it through a day." When I met him, he was taking his medications every two to three hours at an out-of-pocket cost of more than seven hundred dollars per month. Pain and disability seem to shadow his days. As each dose of medicine wanes, aches and limitations descend, he said:

My joints start aching. I get shoulder aches, terribly. And I can't walk at all. I [have] resorted to just getting down and crawling across the floor when I couldn't get someplace. Because you start walking and your legs just won't move. You tend to freeze up. And I swear to myself. [laughs] I would get up and kick something if I could stand up. It is misery. And I know how bad off I am when it's not working. You have to jockey around when you're going to eat. And also to try and juggle the amounts [of medicines]. The trick is to get just the right amount so it takes care of you for that period. If it's too much, you really get the dyskinesia. [If] it's too strong, you can't control the movement. And if it's not enough, the symptoms start coming back and I get cramps in my feet. So you kind of mess with amounts and continue to increase or decrease them, and the times.

This is the panicky feeling. You are out [running an errand]. I was out at the store shopping. And I felt the medicine kind of wearing off and I had a handful of things. And I thought, "Well, the hell with this. I'll get caught in that line up there and I'll fall apart and won't be able to stand up." And so I just left everything on that shelf, wherever it was, and I started getting back to the car. And I knew that I had a limited amount of time before I'd have trouble walking.

His wife interjected, "Tell her about your experience out at the auto shop." Leroy explained that it happened

about noon. I discovered I had a brake light out. At noon I knew my medicine was probably going to start wearing off. And I thought, "Oh, I can get out to the auto parts store and get my bulb and get it back in and have dinner." (I get my medicine before dinner.) So I went out and didn't even take my cane along. And I went into the auto parts store and there was only one customer. And one clerk. And I thought, "Oh, I've got it made. I'll just wait here a minute." But that guy must have had his car being overhauled or something. [laughs]

And I stood there and felt my feet just growing into the floor. I knew I was going to be frozen there. And soon as that person left, I tried to walk forward and my feet wouldn't move. And I'm just struggling and that clerk's standing there watching me. And I tried to put my hand out onto the shelf, to steady me. And I came in contact with a little display that had little key cases and doodads, you know. I felt that thing going over and I took my right hand to steady it and help it out and it just banged the whole thing off. And I slipped and fell and sat right on my butt on the floor with all these little things scattering around me. And the clerk bends way over and says, "Do you need help?" And I thought, "Oh, God." Well, I couldn't tell her. So instead, I still had my bulb in my hand so I said, "Yeah. Do you have a bulb like this one for my brake light?" [laughs] So she went and got it and I got up and—crawled over and got up—and I don't know if she was afraid that I was going to die there. I told her what it was all about, gave her a little synopsis of PD. And she was wiser, and I had my bulb.

It's just an example. You've got to make sure, if you're going somewhere, that you've got this thing timed out where you're going and when you're going to get back. And if you forget to take your medicine, you'll pay for it. [laughs] I was kind of embarrassed, but I saw the humor in that right away, also. Sitting there with these little trinkets setting around me and that clerk bending over me, saying, "Do you need help?" That was partly humorous, yeah. Here I am trying to do my best and knock this whole display off. [laughs]

Outside of the "medication window," the lay term for the frustratingly unpredictable period of time when the medications will "take care of you," the most profound effects of PD on Leroy's life are tied to the medications' side effects. For Leroy, somnolence and freezing shaded the joy he experienced in doing everyday activities. The waking sleepiness makes it almost impossible for him to finish a book or watch a movie. The freezing, an unpredictable inability to move, not only leads him to feel nervous about being out, as the auto parts store episode demonstrates, but also makes it difficult to get to the bathroom in time. He takes a bladder-control medication to help lengthen the time he has to make it to the toilet—a nerve-wracking situation when one is out in public and a potentially embarrassing one wherever he finds himself. Freezing episodes are random and can occur in any situation, but the visual cue of a simple doorway is a common cause. For reasons not well understood, freezing episodes are often triggered by the visual stimuli of doorways, breaks along a wall, or changes in the walking surface. As Leroy explains, "It's almost impossible to hurry. The old phrase, 'The hurrier I am, the behinder I get,' that's it. I just can't hurry."

As I got a better sense of the range of challenges with which Leroy contended on a daily basis, I asked him how he would describe PD.

It's like your own designer disease: "It's all tailored for you—here's yours." It's a disabling disease. It can disable you in a number of ways. Usually, tremor in your hands, difficulty walking, difficulty being fatigued or being able to perform certain tasks that were very easy before. And it's progressive. It will get worse, not better. But it may take years to get worse. [laughs] That's what you keep telling yourself. And generally it's true. It may take years to get worse. . . . When I was in my forties and fifties, I really didn't think that this would happen. You know, I have always kept myself fit, in good physical condition. I thought that old age had its certain drawbacks. You felt old and tired and your joints ached and you got crotchety. But I didn't think of [old age] as being something I was going to experience. Because I had tried to keep myself fit. When this came along, I thought, "It probably is something that I should have expected." PD does come to people in their sixties—which is what I was when I got it. So you reinterpret old age. Sixty-eight isn't nearly as old now as I thought it was. [laughs] But I guess you can *be old*: It's a matter of accepting it also. You accept yourself as being older. But you are constantly looking for a reevaluation of what getting older means. And I guess now getting older means restriction, not being able to do the things that I once did. So the PD has had that effect on that. Of making me reevaluate what being old is.

Coming of Age in Anthropology

Aging is one of the few universals in the human experience, but like all forms of social difference, its meanings and markers are temporally unique sociocultural, historical, and economic moments. Aging is conceived of as an "unpredictable inevitable." We cannot say how or when it will happen, only that inexorably, we will become older. As Howard Stein wrote: "Aging is a vicious affront to the American insistence that the future is limitless, that youth is eternal" (1990, 108). In the United States, two narratives dominate popular concern with aging—efforts to avoid or diminish the effects of biological aging, and ways to care for an aging population that requires a variety of medical, residential, social, and economic services. Such narratives create an ironic tension: Americans at once deny and plan for aging and older age. This tension reveals the intensely negative U.S. bias against human aging and older people. In the discourse of mainstream advertising, aging is a constant struggle to forestall or hide physical and cognitive flaws. The envelopment of aging by senescence raises important questions of meaning and praxis for Americans as they age: If aging is about decline, how can we tell when we are truly sick? And once diagnosed with a chronic disorder, how do we assign causation to emerging somatic phenomena?

Scholarly research on aging reflects the narratives of popular media. Much research on aging validates its importance by citing the public health and social impact produced by an aging population, while it simultaneously strives to combat ageism and the medicalization of yet another aspect of the human life cycle. We know that human life expectancy varies greatly within and among societies, according to people's relative socioeconomic status, gender, reproductive history, and environment. This highlights the important and complex relationship between biological and cultural determinants of aging. In effect, our understanding of the life cycle and human aging is predicated upon exploring these causes of physical, cognitive, and social decline in later life.

Anthropology has a longstanding concern and engagement with how the cultural expression of human diversity is at once a product of local/cultural and universal/physiological forces. The aging process is of particular interest and complexity because we recognize that all peoples as they grow older experience some degree of somatic change, but the interpretation of somatic phenomena is contingent upon the social location of individual older adults. As Gullette (2004) describes it, we are "aged by culture." Cultural practices and beliefs that regard aging as a process of decline invariably shape the interpretation of the body in later life. This interpretive process reveals as much about U.S. notions of aging as it does about the "malignancy" of specific physical or cognitive signs. PD, a disorder whose early symptoms bear a striking resemblance to widely held models of normal older age, presents a unique and thought-provoking case study through which we can examine how culture comes to bear on the experience of the body and ultimately, how older adults' embodiment reflects and produces aging as a parade of unavoidable losses.

The differentiation of what is biological and what is cultural in the aging process continues to drive research into both the experience of aging and social theories of the aging process. Despite anthropology's engagement of elders as keepers of traditional wisdom, anthropological theories of age and aging have received less attention from gerontologists than have theories that draw on sociological or psychological traditions. It has been suggested that U.S. anthropologists are steeped in their own cultural stereotypes regarding the fear of aging and disease and so shy away from its study (Myerhoff 1978). As Christine Fry notes: "Anthropology has a long history of being interested in age, but not in aging or the aged" (1980, 1). The intellectual path forged by Simmons (1945) has been traversed by a number of anthropologists, and a professional organization, the Association for Anthropology and Gerontology, was formed in the early 1970s to promote the development of geroanthropology.

Jennie Keith's (1980) review of this field characterizes it as a tripartite endeavor, and her formulation rings true today. She considers the first category, "old age within anthropology," to include ethnographic works which refer to the knowledge and wisdom of elders as repositories of cultural traditions but which do not focus on the perspectives of elders, per se. The second approach, an "anthropology of age," begins with an understanding of aging as a social and biological process and expands our consideration of the ways in which age is used "as a principle of social organization." The third model, the "anthropology of old age," is represented by texts that explore older adults' lives across cultural or national boundaries. These include ethnographic research on social networks, the development and maintenance of age-segregated communities, and the relationship between cultural beliefs and the aging experience.

More recently, Lawrence Cohen (1994) summarized the state of gerontological anthropology through a critical analysis of its academic tropes. His work serves as an important reminder that academic attention is also a product of culture. Demographic alarmism, righteous indignation, and the trope of ambiguity reveal interesting cultural and epistemological contradictions within the field, he suggests. While many scholars studying aging would profess a desire to improve the plight of elders, the great irony is that "a discipline [gerontology] is articulated to demonstrate the normality of old age by segregating its study and treatment from that of young and middle adulthood" (142). Cohen suggests three directions for geroanthropology: "a phenomenological focus on experience, embodiment, and identity; a critical focus on the rationalities and hegemonies through which aging is experienced and presented; and an interpretive focus on the relevance of the ethnographer's age to the forms of knowledge produced" (152). These areas represent growing attention to the locating of cultural "scripts" regarding the aging process in the individual body and the maturation of interpretive theory concerning narratives and their construction of self and reality.

Cohen's is the most recent major review of geroanthropology, and since the time of that essay, 1994, a number of important ethnographic works examining aging and elders have been published. Major themes in contemporary geroanthropology are the socioeconomic and health care issues associated with aging populations (Albert 2004; Le Navenec and Bridges 2005); issues of identity, self-hood, suffering, and embodiment in particular age-related disorders (Black 2006; Black and Rubinstein 2000, 2004; Leibing and Cohen 2006; McLean 2006); elders' subcultural experiences and the meaning of retirement (Savishinsky 2000); long-term care and congregate housing as cultural and medical phenomena (Ball et al. 2005; Stafford 2003; Zimmerman, Sloane, and Eckert 2001); crosscultural perspectives on death and dying (Francis, Kellaher, and Neophytou 2005); biocultural perspectives on human aging (Crews 2003; Ice 2005); and cross-cultural variation in grandparenting (Albert and Cattell 1994; Armstrong 2005; Cliggett 2005). More broadly speaking, attention to aging by anthropologists has focused productively on the medicalization of aging, the social production of the aging body, and the importance of narrative to understanding these processes. Much of this work has been conducted by medical anthropologists studying aging.

Medical Anthropology and Interpretive Approaches
to Aging and Sickness

Medical anthropology is at the heart of anthropological grappling with the universality of the human experience. As a subdiscipline of anthropology, medical anthropology focuses on the interactions between biology and culture (Foster and Anderson 1978) and is predicated upon the idea that medical events are at once biological and cultural (Romanucci-Ross, Moerman, and Tancredi 1991). Anthropologists have examined this interaction through such examples as dementia (Herskovits 1995; Leibing and Cohen 2006), mental illness (Kleinman 1988b), pain (Finkler 1994), the placebo effect (Moerman 2002), and childbirth (Davis-Floyd 2003; Martin 1987). These examples demonstrate the ways in which natural science, whose cultural authority invokes an acultural vantage, is fully embedded in larger cultural systems of power, inequality, and meaning. They highlight the complexity of differentiating between biology and culture in the experience of sickness and point to our reliance upon scientific knowledge as both a measure and a product of a cultural system that privileges science (Latour 2000). Medical anthropology may have begun as a comparative endeavor, examining cross-cultural variation in the definitions and treatment of sickness, but it has come to integrate a self-reflexivity exploring how humans create meaning from somatic experience. This study of meaning making includes the perspectives of the sick, their healers, and the larger community, and the perspectives of these disparate stakeholders can be explicated by incorporating multiple theoretical constructs: the disease/illness framework, explanatory models, illness narratives, embodiment, suffering, and the life course perspective. Linking these historical, emerging, and interdisciplinary approaches to the study of disease works to build a framework for understanding the experience of both aging and chronic illness in a new light. Drawing on the strengths of each demonstrates how thinking of a disorder such as PD as a *condition* can increase our compassion and understanding of both particular disorders and age-related change.

The Disease/Illness Framework

The disease/illness framework is a construct that aims to identify variation in the interpretation of "sickness," a term encompassing both disease and illness, by differentiating between the perspective of the sick and that of healers. As Eisenberg defines it: "To state it flatly, patients suffer 'illness'; physicians diagnose and treat 'diseases.' Let me make clear the distinction I intend: illnesses are experiences of disvalued changes in states of being and social function; diseases, in the scientific paradigm of modern medicine, are abnormalities in the structure and function of body organs and systems" (1977, 11). Or, as Kleinman phrases it, illness is the "cultural dressing" laid upon disease (1988a). The disease/illness model is useful to think with, allowing us to recognize the dissonance between what patients may experience and the validation of that experience by healers. Yet, while the construct can demonstrate power relations in sickness, it seems to simultaneously imply that the disease perspective is objective and the illness subjective. Staiano (1986) also notes that the disease/illness distinction reflects and perpetuates the mind/body dualism of biomedicine, whereby illness is equated with the patient's standpoint and experience, firmly positioning this perspective as the lesser of two knowledges. In defense of the disease/illness dichotomy, Lupton argues: "This definition, of course, does not necessarily imply that disease is an objective state, for as scholars from the social constructionist perspective argue, the categorizing of disease is influenced by the social, historical and political context as is the definition of illness" (1994, 93). And Kleinman points out that neither disease nor illness categories refer to "things," but rather to different, and differently privileged, vantage points on the same moment in sickness (1978; 1988a).

Talcott Parsons's (1979) work on the sick role illustrates the site of power in this dialectic quite clearly. The medical practitioner has the power to grant the sick role to an ailing patient. Whatever the patient's experience of pain, disability, or illness might be, this experience must be validated by a health care practitioner in order for a patient to *legitimately* be sick (Kleinman 1977). This conceptualization of the illness experience as primarily one of deviance seems best suited to the understanding of acute conditions, where the acceptable time frame for the role is clear (Foster and Anderson 1978).

The relative power of these social locations is determined by the overarching cultural system that defines biomedicine's position as acultural and objective and patients' perspectives as mere "beliefs." Medicine can be understood as a system of social control whereby those who have the power to draw boundaries around physical experiences and label them diseases and those who have the authority to acknowledge symptoms as illness and translate illness into disease have social power (Crawford 1984; Kunstadter 1974; Taussig 1980). However, despite the authority afforded physicians and biomedical researchers, medical anthropological research has demonstrated that scientific knowledge is produced within a cultural context by social actors who possess varying degrees of credibility—including medical experts, the media, activists, governmental organizations and the public (Epstein 1999; Koenig and Marshall 2004). Thus, biomedical practitioners are no longer the silent object to which all patient/subjects are compared, but also culturally situated subjects worthy of scrutiny (Mendehlson 1974).

Explanatory Models

In considering medicine and its practitioners as cultural actors imbued with meaning and authority, medical anthropologists have developed and adopted a series of conceptual tools with which to investigate power, meaning, and the processes by which culture shapes the lived experience of the body. Arthur Kleinman's articulate and popular explanatory model (EM) framework was one of the first attempts to operationalize medical anthropological inquiry. EMs represent how illness is defined, perceived, and treated by practitioners, as well as how patients can legitimately respond to symptoms of disease. There are five key features of an EM—etiology, onset of symptoms, pathophysiology, course of illness, and treatment (Kleinman 1977, 1978). These components help us to understand why patients behave the way they do when they are sick. Patient-held EMs are temporally and culturally specific; "explanatory models are not ways of thinking or systems of thought but practical statements about particular illness experiences" (Kleinman 1981, 375). The strength of EMs comes from their emphasis on situated, localized meanings (Farmer and Good 1991). They are products of individuals, of specific illness incidents, and of unique temporal moments. The meanings of EMs lie in the relationship of the individuals to society, in the context of their sickness, and in the relationships between patients and health care providers. EMs focus on the dyadic relationship between patient and provider as the central location of meaning and importance (Kleinman 1988b).

Explanatory models are well employed as a starting point for the study of the sickness experience. Through an EM, we can obtain a snapshot of the outgrowth of the cultural production of somatic experience. However, EMs may be better suited to the study of acute than of chronic illness episodes, as "the differing explanatory models offered by a patient and his social networks and his healers are incomplete, mutually contradictory, and redundant, especially for an ongoing illness crisis where the outcome is still uncertain" (Blumhagen 1981, 338). Thus, while we can learn much about the meaning of illness through the comparison of sufferers' EMs, the temporal nature of chronic illness makes EMs especially fragmentary.

Illness Narratives and the Life Course Perspective

If EMs provide a synchronic view of sickness, how can we hope to access the diachronic *process* of a sickness experience? We can begin by considering disease and illness as forms of communication (Lupton 1994). "The experience called illness, the signs and symptoms as they are reported and expressed, the process whereby such signs are interpreted, are all semiotic phenomena, subject to semiotic interpretation" (Staiano 1986, 2). Rich exploration of this semiotic communication is found in academic discourse on illness narratives, the practice of embodiment, and the relationships shared by social actors engaged in the sickness experience. Illness narratives are a sort of social medical history through which anthropologists elicit from sufferers an extensive, open-ended articulation of their experience. As medical sociologist Conrad describes them: "Relevant questions include how people first notice 'something is wrong' and what it means to them, what kinds of theories and explanations they develop to make sense of these unusual events, what they do about their problem, how they come to seek medical care and with what concerns and expectations, what impact diagnosis has on them, and how they cope with a medical label and managing regimes" (1990, 1260).

Illness narratives focus on the *process* of becoming sick (or in this case, aged) rather than on just the *product* of such cultural processes (Keith and Kertzer 1984). Illness narratives contextualize the illness experience within the life course experience of the afflicted, thus moving us closer to an understanding of how sickness is produced (Young 1982). In doing so, the illness narrative approach also decenters the primacy or dominance of the disease-oriented medical perspective. Sickness alters identity, and sufferers use narrative to reconstitute selfhood (Gubrium and Holstein 1999; Riessman 1993, 2001). Attention to illness narratives can provide a larger framework for making sense of how sociocultural factors come to shape the life course and situates the current moment as an active and evolving artifact (Gerhardt 1990; Myerhoff and Simic 1978).

Illness narratives are especially poignant in regard to chronic illness, as diagnosis is often related as a moment of "biographical disruption" (Becker 1997; Bury 1982; Riessman 1993). While illness narratives are constructed in sociohistorical and biographical moments, they are at the same time longer and broader perspectives on the sufferer's experience of illness. Illness narratives position social experiences at the center of inquiry and demonstrate how people live with chronic illness. These extended autobiographical stories are ways by which sufferers, through the veil of culture, construct meaning from biographical and embodied experiences. More simply, the body is the "existential ground of culture" (Csordas 1990), and illness narratives are one way in which social knowledge can be communicated (Lock 1993).

Such a perspective is echoed in the groundswell of support for the life course perspective within gerontology. Gerontologists, long concerned with elders' quality of life, have become more invested in examining the ways in which lifelong variables such as employment history, marital satisfaction, social status, and health status can direct individuals' aging trajectory toward or away from what has come to be called "successful aging" (see Rowe and Kahn 1998). In the phenomenological and social constructivist paradigms, scholars have given increasingly vocal support to the value of a life course vantage for understanding elders' narratives (Stamm et al. 2008). Meaning in later life is derived in part from lifelong social, economic, biological, and psychological factors that shape the experience of older age. This premise rings familiar in medical anthropology and sociology, where the connection between the social and the biological has long been established. However, the discovery of narrative in gerontology has only more recently been linked to such discourse. While aging is certainly not a process of inevitable suffering and sickness, our recognition of the relationships between chronic illness and aging, and of how narratives can explicate them, is gaining prominence.

The Body, Embodiment, and Suffering

While the diachronic perspective afforded by illness narratives can demonstrate how somatic experience is created, it also may demonstrate sufferers' embodied experiences, as "the body unlocks a moral universe that often escapes social (symbolic) discourse" (Van Wolputte 2004, 260). Anthropological attention to the body is long lived and varied, and there are several excellent reviews of this literature to orient scholars to its discursive threads (see in particular Lock 1993; Strathern 2004; Van Wolputte 2004). My use of the word "body" refers to the material, biological entity in which we find ourselves more or less inextricably ensconced. By "embodiment," I mean the process by which we (1) mediate the relationship of the self and the somatic; and (2) interpret, understand, and create meaning for ourselves in the context of particular cultural experiences, such as aging or sickness. As Van Wolputte puts it: "This contemporary body-self is fragmentary, often incoherent and inconsistent, precisely because it arises from contradictory and paradoxical experiences, tensions, and conflicts that have one thing in common: They are real, that is, experienced. Therefore, the anthropology of the body focuses no longer on the abstract or ideal(ized) body, but on those moments during which the body and bodiliness are questioned and lose their self-evidence and on the experience or threat of finiteness, limitations, transience and vulnerability" (2004, 263).

This approach to the body and embodiment draws upon the works of Scheper-Hughes and Lock (1987), Lock (1993), and Csordas (1990; 1993a,b). Using EMs, illness narratives, and participant observation I provide a window into how the aging body comes to be embodied in particular ways, as seen from varying levels of analysis. In this sense my work uses the notion of embodiment as a way to operationalize the integration of Scheper-Hughes and Lock's "three bodies"—the individual body, "the phenomenological sense of the lived experience of the body-self"; the social body, "the representational uses of the body as a natural symbol with which to think about nature, society, and culture"; and the body politic, "the regulation, surveillance, and control of bodies (individual and collective)" (1987, 7). Integration of the three bodies constitutes a holistic project and a model that has the potential to break from what Turner (1993) identifies as the two "traps" in body discourse, whereby the body is either reified as a "bounded individual," or the material realities of the body are eschewed in favor of a conceptual, discursive body. In formulating the body as a set of nested vantage points or sites of meaning making, integration of the three bodies recognizes the experiential and structural aspects of sickness (Kaufman 1988).

As participants in a wider culture, human beings both *have* bodies and *are* bodies; accordingly, embodiment—the experience of the body—is integrally connected to conceptions of identity and self (Hockey and James 2003). Embodiment, then, offers a way to access an interstitial space—the place between perception and the production of understanding—a space made more visible in instances such as illness where the body's relationship to the self is highlighted (Csordas 1993b, 2002; Faircloth et al. 2004; Svenaeus 2000). "This approach to embodiment begins from the methodological postulate that the body is not an object to be studied in relation to culture, but is to be considered the subject of culture, or in other words as the existential ground of culture" (Csordas 2002, 58). Embodiment is one way that individuals make sense of somatic phenomena in a specific sociocultural setting, and the concept can be employed to gain a better understanding of the illness perspective and the underlying rationale for people's health-related behaviors.

Because age, like gender, is accomplished through performance, the embodiment of aging is an inescapable component of cultural reality and one that is often accomplished via the somatic body (Laz 2003). The aged body is an outward and objective one that is shaped by experience and constitutes a "project of interpretive practice" (Gubrium and Holstein 2003). Aging bodies, however, cannot always enact agency, as elders who live with a chronic illness can attest (Laz 2003). Attention to aged bodies is nothing new, but an attention to the aging body as a site of meaning production has only recently emerged. Aging is a universal process that has stimulated fruitful discussion of the universality of human biology, but few scholars have investigated how the aging body and the concept of embodiment are together complicit in the cultural production of aging (Faircloth 2003a). A focus on embodiment highlights the interplay between biological and social aging, and may demonstrate "how people experience the body as a mundane entity and the process by which they give meaning to it" (Faircloth 2003b, 6). The aging body poses a unique opportunity to further our understanding of embodiment because of its outward markers. The body is a public surface (Strathern 2004), and both older age and PD are displayed in overt physicality, apprehendable to others.

A phenomenological approach such as this must keep the biological nature of human bodies, disease, and aging in focus, lest it risk negating this dimension of being or reduce experience to symbolism and power (Good 1994). It must strive to maintain a balance between understanding the embodiment of aging in chronic disease as a function of somatic maladies and viewing these maladies in a context of social suffering. Social suffering is the recognition of the forces in play that produce an inextricable web in which people experience their individual life course (Kleinman, Das, and Lock 1997). Suffering is an all-encompassing experience and "a visceral awareness of the self's vulnerability to be broken or diminished at any time and in many ways" (Black and Rubinstein 2004, S23). Maintaining an awareness of this dimension of human development grounds the study of aging in a respectful humanistic stance. With such an awareness, we can explain the myriad social forces that situate elders in their particular life worlds without exoticizing their sorrows and challenges or further stigmatizing their marked bodies.

Conditions, a Special Case of Sickness

Inasmuch as illness narratives can convey sufferers' autobiographical process of becoming sick, in the case of chronic disorders sufferers' reluctance to identify themselves as sick limits the utility of the dichotomy. Corbin raises this issue in her discussion of the sickness experience: "So, I wondered, if one can have a chronic illness/condition and not consider oneself to be ill, what does it mean to be ill?" (2003, 257). In my study of aging with PD, I learned that while sufferers recognize the progressive, incurable nature of the disorder, describing PD as a disease, they do not identify themselves as sick. A few people categorized PD as a disability, and others considered it to be a layer of their identity—somewhat proudly referring to themselves as "Parkys" or "Parkinsonians." But for many sufferers PD was simply embodied as a *condition* with which they lived and aged.

Calling something a condition is a way to situate the liminal existence of chronic disorders, such as stroke recovery, multiple sclerosis, or diabetes, that leave sufferers in an in-between place somewhere between the sick and the well. Conditions may represent a third state of being in the sickness experience, one that is positioned between illness and disease. Used in the colloquial sense, a condition is a limitation or restriction placed upon action and experience. The term is commonly used to refer to disabling somatic phenomena that influence the sufferer's mode of being in the world. Considering PD as a condition helps us to recognize the changing nature of patients' medical knowledge in the United States. In today's media-saturated environment, many PD sufferers access, interpret, and internalize biomedical models of the disorder. This emerging relationship to biomedical knowledge moves them further away from an archetypal illness vantage point and closer to a biomedical disease perspective. However, sufferers' explanations for how PD functions, where it resides in the body, and its causes remain varied and individual. In this way, viewing PD as a condition acknowledges a dialogic relationship between illness and disease and responds to the ways in which increased access to medical knowledge has altered the power dynamic between patients and practitioners in contemporary biomedical encounters.

While PD certainly poses unique challenges to personhood, identity, and health maintenance, it bears similarities to other chronic disorders that make the condition concept a potentially valuable tool with which to consider embodiment. As conditions on the body and embodiment, chronic illnesses share the temporal framework of an interminable sickness experience: They offer an uncertain prognosis, they compel lifelong medical management, they foment substantive reflection on sufferers' identity, and they require adjustments to housing, travel, and other aspects of social life.

Kathy Charmaz's body of work on chronic illness illustrates this commonality across such conditions quite clearly. She argues that suffering in chronic illness is linked to a loss of selfhood, and that part of this loss stems from the inability of an individual's life course metric to now adequately assess ability and positive self-concept (Charmaz 1983). This shift in metric is underscored by Western culture's definition of the increments as independence and self-reliance. Thus, as we lose independence, we consequently lose identity (Charmaz 1983). Furthermore, in this loss of selfhood, the blame and shame associated with decreased abilities fall within the sphere of the individual. As chronic illness sufferers learn to manage their ever-changing abilities and strive to overcome the limitations of their autobiographical metric, their suffering is increased by the social obligation to downplay disability and demonstrate self-control. The chronically ill are often constricted by social mores as much as they are by their disorder (Charmaz 1983). The unpredictability of chronic illness increases the challenge of a public performance of normalcy, compelling many sufferers to withdraw into private spaces and lose another measure of ability—the social context of identity (Charmaz 1983).

Charmaz complements Corbin and Strauss (1988) in that she too positions chronic illness as biographical disruption (1991). Chronic illnesses dislocate autobiographical narratives. They strive but fail to fit into an acute care, illness-oriented model of embodiment. Sufferers adhere to treatment regimens in the hope that good compliance will yield a cure or remission, and they expect that a diagnosis will be accompanied by a prognosis that ends their somatic questioning (Charmaz 1991). Instead, what chronic illness sufferers find is that being ill requires time, accommodation, and attention. They must live their lives around the preestablished, though unpredictable, demands of illness constraints and needs. Sufferers are socially obligated to control symptoms and their sequelae for fear of embarrassment or ostracism, and they begin to measure the quality of their days by the intrusiveness of their disability (Charmaz 1991).

Charmaz's perspective in *Good Days, Bad Days* is consistent with the conditions model I propose. In particular, she notes that older adults are socially expected to live with illness-related constraints and to view such disorders not as illness but *as part of life*: "No longer can people add illness to the structure of their lives; instead they must reconstruct their lives upon illness" (1991, 76).

Other recent work on embodiment in chronic illness also supports the notion of conditions as the embodiment of the in-between. Öhman, Söderberg, and Lundman's (2003) study of illness narratives from cancer, rheumatoid arthritis, kidney disease, and neurological disorder sufferers identified three central themes in their experiences. Sufferers experience the body as a hindrance or a barrier to their independence, they suffered from social isolation and felt that they lived between the two poles of hope and despair, and they sought meaning and explanation for their disorder by struggling to attain mastery at whatever level of ability they could now achieve. Sufferers reported that they felt as if they were only half a person: Individuals possessed the same inner desires and will, but only half their historical abilities. Faircloth, Boylstein, Rittman, and Young's (2004) study of stroke survivors also speaks to the performative work of appearing in control, healthy, or normal. Stroke sufferers in their study managed identity by objectifying the disability and separating it from the body, by enacting small daily tasks to test the body's compliance with personal will, and by coming to consider the body a "biographically informed phenomena." The inability of the body to respond to the mind's command contributed to the utility of objectifying impairments, and sufferers demonstrated this in part by speaking aloud to their bodies, as if they were separate and will-laden entities of their own (84).

A small study of women's experiences with multiple sclerosis (MS) also identified several strategies for managing the disconnect between historical and current ability, between being well and being sick. Reynolds and Prior (2003) found that, as in PD, women with MS experience mobility problems and fatigue that can contribute to premature retirement; their motor impairments may lead others to wonder if they are drugged or inebriated; and the unpredictability of relapsing-remitting symptoms and prognosis make it difficult for others to maintaining empathy and understanding Women with MS manage this uneasy social location by being proactive about health promotion, striving to maintain role continuity by adapting meaningful roles to fit their current somatic ability, and pursuing disease advocacy to improve sufferers' social position and quality of life. Similarly to PD, the "pacing" or adjustments women make to this condition are experienced along a continuum of "healthy adjustment" and "giving in." Adaptations are framed as a way to gain or maintain mastery and identity, the authors found, but women continued to negotiate how much activity they should expect to squeeze into a good day, their positive coping did not eradicate anger or frustration, and the shame and ostracism of disabling environments were constantly being negotiated.

Diabetics must also navigate the space between sickness and wellness, according to Ingadottir and Halldorsdottir (2008). As one subject in a recent qualitative study commented: "[Diabetes] is not a disease, unless you make it a disease. It's just a certain lifestyle which I did not choose" (610). Adherence issues in diabetes self-care are a major public health issue, and like PD sufferers, diabetics often tailor their interminable medication regimen to individual desires and goals to offset the negative impact such medication reliance has upon identity. Diabetics in Ingadottir and Halldorsdottir's study established identity continuity by obtaining knowledge and mastery of the disorder and striving to live as they had prior to diagnosis and as much "outside" disease management guidelines as possible. As do PD sufferers, diabetics want to be independent and self-determined. Yet gaining autonomy via self-knowledge is ongoing, because knowledge is always partial and becomes more so as the disorder progresses, the body's response to medications changes, and one's own goals and aspirations change, the researchers found. Diabetic sufferers in this study identified a measure of autonomy by viewing themselves as healthy and avoiding drawing attention to the condition. Thus, diabetics may elect to take blood-sugar readings or have snacks in private, while PD sufferers take extra medication to ensure functioning or hide their shaking hands under their arms or in their pockets.

Across these chronic disorders and others, it is clear that suffering arises from both somatic and social sites, and that the severity of one's suffering is intrinsically related to autobiographical narrative and social context. As Ironside et al. (2003) argue, to understand the experience of such disorders we must move away from our preoccupation with functional status and symptomatic relief to a perspective that situates such impairments within a meaningful social and historical milieu. Biographical disruption remains a compelling stance from which to view the impact of chronic illness upon sufferers' identities and social experiences, but it at times implies that individuals' biographical narratives have a predetermined trajectory, which, when interrupted, foments a process of identity maintenance and reconstruction. Certainly, suffering arises from the inability to fulfill an expected or valued social role (Aujoulat, Luminet, and Deccache 2007), yet sufferers seek an alternative discourse to reflect their almost healthy but not quite ill status.

As Frank writes: "Suffering is what makes illness worth studying, just as illness is what makes health care a topic of concern" (2001, 353). Suffering can occur in the absence of sickness (Black and Rubinstein 2004; Frank 2001), and biographical revision may be part of identity maintenance in late modernity (Williams 2000). In fact, as Williams (2000) points out, biographical disruption is based on an assumption that the body vis-à-vis identity is comprehensible until a certain age. In contrast, conditions can be understood as a special practice of embodiment, the process by which sociocultural beliefs concerning the normal and anticipated processes of aging come to be internalized, interpreted, and experienced by individual older adults. Viewing PD as a condition, as a state of embodiment between disease and illness, emphasizes the complexities inherent in its treatment and demonstrates the importance of social context in understanding the aging experience.

Parkinson's Disease as a Case Study

PD disease affords a unique opportunity to explore the embodiment of aging for a variety of overlapping factors. The number of young onset PD cases is increasing in industrialized nations, but PD remains a disorder that primarily affects older adults. Organic disease precedes clinical manifestations of symptoms, which generally become troublesome and noticeable in the sixth decade of life. The early symptoms of slowness, stiff movement, and stooped posture are thus not only the sort of somatic signs that many of us would consider benign aches and pains, but these changes present at the same time of life when sufferers are beginning the transition from parent to grandparent, from full-time paid employment to part-time work or retirement, and from adult to older adult.

The progressive nature of PD adds to the complexity of allocating embodiment to disease or older age. As the disorder increases in severity and changes from a lateral nuisance to global mobility impairment, it produces outwardly visible, stigmatizing signs. Embarrassment drives a desire to avoid unfamiliar social settings, which in turn intensifies sufferers' feelings that they are losing control of their bodies and lives. Daily reminders of limitations, be they mobility problems, disabling environments, or only partly effective medications, reflect the power of the disorder to shape one's sense of the future. Older age is no longer envisioned as a possible decline, but as an inevitable one. Decisions concerning insurance, travel, housing, advanced directives, or support services are made in the context not only of increasing age but also of aging with a condition. This condition is the gamble, the evaluation of likelihoods, that can overshadow life or overcome efforts to maintain continuity of self.

In the case of PD, the experience of somatic change is trumped by the knowledge of disease progression, the ubiquity of age-related change, and the increasing alienation of the once-predictable body from the self. As the disease becomes more severe and the medications less able to confer control, the relationship between one's body and one's self is mediated by an ever-fluctuating set of conditions. Progression is inevitable but unpredictable, and comparison to other PD sufferers is of limited utility in evaluating the normalcy of one's individual case. As Leroy phrases it in the introduction to this chapter, "It's like your own designer disease: 'It's all tailored for you—here's yours.'"

Public recognition of PD has increased dramatically through the advocacy efforts of celebrity sufferers like Michael J. Fox and Muhammad Ali, but recognition of PD's global impact on sufferers' social worlds has only recently emerged in public health and academic literatures. From a public health standpoint, PD is a particularly important disorder due to its increasing prevalence and its consumption of medical resources. PD compels expensive and life-long medical intervention and is more frequent in rural populations, known to be the most difficult to serve. Yet a majority of research on PD remains divorced from the social location of its experience.

Parkinson's Disease: An Overview

PD is a progressive neurological condition most common in adults aged sixty or older. PD prevalence is estimated at 1 percent of persons aged fifty and older

(Duvoisin and Sage 1996). The underlying pathology is generally understood by neurologists to be related to the death of dopamine-producing neurons in the substantia nigra, part of the midbrain; however, the ultimate cause of PD remains unknown. The decrease in dopaminergic neuronal activity negatively affects motor performance, and disease progression can lead to severe motor impairment. For the majority of sufferers, PD first shows up as slowed movement, stooped posture, slowed gait, and a mild to moderate tremor on one side of the body. The onset of symptoms can be slow, but the rate of progression varies tremendously, from two to thirty years (Curtis and McDonald 1998). Progression can be linked to a number of related problems, including persistent fatigue, shuffling gait, slouch, mumbled speech, decreased ability to demonstrate facial affect, urinary urgency, visual disturbances, micrographia, or sleep disturbances (Duvoisin and Sage 1996; Fitzsimmons and Bunting 1993). In the later stages incontinence, neuropsychiatric disorders (such as depression or anxiety), dysphagia (difficulty swallowing), and postural instability that can cause injurious falls may appear (Curtis and McDonald 1998; Friesen and Mateer 2001; Monguio 2001). It is estimated that about 20 percent of PD patients also show signs of dementia (Curtis and McDonald 1998; Fitzsimmons and Bunting 1993; Woodruff-Pak 1997). To underscore PD's heterogeneity, one sufferer may have had PD for fifteen years and experience little disruption to their life, whereas another person may go from a light tremor to severe disability over the course of five years.

Older adults and general practitioners both can mistake the early signs of PD for normal aging, as was the case for Leroy (see also Pinder 1990). Thus, many older adults live with unremitting symptoms for several years before learning that PD is the source of their problems. The diagnostic moment is very much imbued with a sense of arrival and uncertainty, as sufferers are temporarily satisfied to have a name for their condition, only to be deeply dismayed by their prognosis. Life after diagnosis can become a thorough and profound reevaluation of identity and ability. Virtually all PD sufferers take medication to relieve their symptoms, and as the disorder progresses, the number, cost, and complexity of pharmacological regimens increase exponentially.

Such diagnostic tools as blood tests, magnetic resonance imagery, or X-rays are currently of little utility to PD diagnosis. PD is a clinical diagnosis arrived at when patients, usually "of a certain age," present with three signs—tremor, rigidity, and bradykinesia, slowness in the execution of movement (Duvoisin and Sage 1996). Diagnosis is confirmed when the patient responds positively to carbidopa-levodopa, a medication that increases the amount of dopamine in the brain and subsequently improves motor function. Carbidopa-levodopa does not cure PD nor does it slow disease progression. Discovered in the 1960s, carbidopa-levodopa is a mainstay treatment for PD symptoms, but it is also produces its own impairments. After seven to ten years on the medication, many users develop dyskinesia, freezing, and the end of dose phenomena (also known as the on/off syndrome) (Curtis and McDonald 1998). When this sensitivity and decreased efficacy occur, sufferers must work to find a balance between being frozen, unable to move, and dyskinesia, where they experience undesirable movements. Due to medication side effects such as hallucinations, psychosis, or anxiety, sufferers are sometimes forced to choose between motor and cognitive performance (Fitzsimmons and Bunting 1993). Compliance with medication regimes can be difficult, and as PD progresses, the medications become less effective in controlling increasingly severe symptoms (Duvoisin and Sage 1996). In addition, the medications may cost upwards of three hundred dollars per month (Fitzsimmons and Bunting 1993).

Parkinson's symptoms affect every aspect of daily life. Sufferers can have difficulty navigating bathrooms, turning over in bed, walking, and eating (Brod, Mendelsohn, and Roberts 1998). Many PD sufferers fear that they will lose their driver's license and so self-limit their driving to daytime hours and short distances. Gait problems caused by tremor, bradykinesia, postural instability, or stooped posture dramatically increase their risk of falling and sustaining serious injury. PD-related motor problems can become quite severe and contribute to decreased mobility and social engagement. Cognitive symptoms, such as an overall slowed cognitive function, memory loss, or impaired executive function cause patients and their spouses alike much frustration and distress.

The disorder's symptoms, its diagnosis, treatment, and impact on daily life all precipitate a considerable decline in sufferers' quality of life. This has not gone unremarked in the medical literature, and there are several well-validated PD-specific quality of life measures that demonstrate the degree to which PD sufferers' lives are impacted by the disorder (Jenkinson, Fitzpatrick, and Peto 1999). However, much of the attention paid to PD has concentrated upon the management of symptoms to the detriment of cultural or psychosocial issues (Fitzsimmons and Bunting 1993). This has led Koplas and colleagues to call for a new research agenda, asserting that, "in order for the medical community to optimize management of patients with PD, health care providers need to look beyond medical treatments for specific symptoms and ask how PD affects an individual's overall quality of life" (1999, M197).

It is clear from the sizable autobiographical literature on living with PD that the disorder profoundly impacts the social lives of patients and their families (see appendix B for a bibliography of such patient narratives). Academic writing on the lived experience of PD is scant but rich. Ruth Pinder's (1990, 1992) ethnographic work in England investigated patient and physician responses to PD diagnosis. She describes an interesting disconnect between these actors in the sickness encounter. Physicians, who are trained to diagnosis disease, find a sense of coherence upon arriving at a PD diagnosis and may view it as "not too bad" in the scope of neurological illnesses. Among patients, a PD diagnosis intensifies feelings of being old and feeling cheated by life. In Pinder's words: "The idea of slowly disintegrating, or gradually losing control over one's mental faculties and bodily functions, of being helpless and dependent in a culture which places a high premium on self-reliance and independence aroused intense dread in some patients" (1992, 17). Further, the extensive medication regime negatively impacted patients, "emphasizing the fact that they were no longer in control over their own bodies" (19). A sociological study conducted in the Netherlands examines the influence of PD on selfhood and identity (Nijhof 1995). Participants in this study felt stigmatized by the outward signs of the disorder. They expressed a fear of being perceived by others as intoxicated or mentally ill, which led some patients to withdraw from public spaces and spend more time at home. This was also found by Fitzsimmons and Bunting, who comment: "Often patients will express embarrassment due to their gait disturbance and verbalize a realistic fear that others will assume they have a substance abuse problem" (1993, 811). More recently, Bramley and Eatough (2005) conducted a phenomenological study of PD based on three interviews with a woman in her sixties living with PD. Their interpretation of her narratives focused on the daily struggles she endured in trying to use her unpredictable and less functional body, as well as her process of identity transformation.

The Embodiment of Aging in the Case of Parkinson's Disease

The overarching question guiding my study of PD and aging was, How do cultural perceptions of aging as inexorable decline influence the experiences of older adults living with PD, a disorder whose signs mimic commonly held perceptions of normal aging? Admittedly, this question is to an extent unanswerable, for, as discussed, our ideas about biology are always products of cultural moments. Further, ethnographic research is not well equipped to delineate the borders between what is normal and what might be termed pathological in the aging process. As a feminist and medical geroanthropologist, my aim, by examining the embodiment of aging in the case of PD, is to elucidate the repercussions of conflating aging with senescence.

Considering PD as a condition *of* and *on* older age, I set out to learn how PD sufferers come to make sense of aging and the body while living with a progressive disorder. Drawing on pilot research and the extant PD literature, I undertook fieldwork with the premise that, because PD is sometimes at first taken to be normal old age, sufferers' age at onset would influence their perception of somatic phenomena. I theorized that the younger the age of onset, the more likely one would be to seek medical advice for one's symptoms. I also thought that the more outwardly visible and stigmatizing signs of PD, such as tremor and gait problems, would be more likely to compel someone to seek care than those considered more benign, such as slowness or stooped posture. I began the study focusing on PD diagnosis as an endpoint of interest, and I spent a great deal of time talking with people about their diagnostic trajectory—the thoughts, events, and random chances that drew them toward the discovery that they had PD. As is often the case in ethnography, the story that I expected to hear was not the one communicated in the narratives I collected.

When PD sufferers or caregivers asked me what my study was about, and wondered what in the world anthropology could have to do with PD, I explained that being sick is a cultural phenomenon. They understood my interest in PD as a disease of older age, but they would sometimes ask, "Is this study about old age or is it about PD?" We would share a laugh as I returned their question with one of my own—"What's worse, being old or having PD?" The inextricability of aging and PD came to the fore when I began to realize that relationships among diagnostic trajectories, the interpretation of early PD symptoms, and sufferers' disease duration, gender, number of medications taken, decade of life, and poor health status were not in evidence.

Ironically, I began this project as a study of "becoming ill" and came to recognize that embodiment was more about "being ill" (Pierret 2003). Yes, PD is sometimes mistaken for older age, and this interpretation meaningfully reflects the persistence with which many Americans equate aging with physical decline. PD sufferers' diagnostic trajectories detail many instances of such ageism, both internal and external. But, the larger story *begins* at diagnosis, when people expect to arrive at resolution and find only ambiguity. In characterizing this larger narrative and sifting through the heterogeneity of individuals for broader patterns of meaning, it became clear that the embodiment of aging is made evident in relief: PD is a condition that accelerates, mediates, and obscures aging. Despite their age at disease onset, sufferers experience the embodiment of PD through their current age.

The experience of growing older is imbued by sufferers' status as sick and the knowledge that they possess a disabling and progressive disorder. Embarrassing symptoms, the use of and dependence upon medications, stooped posture, expressionless face, and reliance upon assistive devices contribute to an acceleration of aging. For people with these symptoms, having PD increased the speed with which they had to adjust to anticipated age-related changes. In this sense, when sufferers say that they feel *old* before their time, they are at once reflecting and reproducing the embodiment of aging as an inexorable decline. The symptoms of PD that overlap with stereotypical markers of older age cause sufferers to wonder if they are just getting old or if something is *really* wrong. This mode of being is characterized by *mediation*. Such narratives struggle to tease apart aging and PD in an effort to mark disease progression and to be able to suss out which somatic changes might be socially acceptable to discuss. Having a diagnosis gives some PD sufferers license to discuss personal problems that others might otherwise interpret as complaining. PD can produce a mode of being in older age that serves to *obscure* age-related changes. These narratives emphasize the ways in which a PD diagnosis is used to explain all the changes in someone's life. Sufferers unconsciously use PD as a covering term for their aging, attributing their retirement or relocation decisions to the disorder. Similarly, according to PD sufferers, physicians are blind to other explanations or comorbidities when they see a PD diagnosis on the chart.

When these categories are applied to individual illness narratives, age emerges as an important variable of interest. Each decade of life is associated with a particular mode of being. Sufferers in their sixties regarded PD as a condition which sped up biological and social aging. Sufferers in their seventies described PD as a mediator of aging processes: They experienced suffering when they found that they could not distinguish between normal aging and disease progression. Those sufferers in their eighties and older embodied PD as a stand-in for aging. Their experience of late life was predominantly one of disease and disorder and much less about aging per se. As the remainder of this book aims to show, elders' experiences of PD reflect and reproduce the idea that aging is about decline, but in ways relative to their individual case and their particular location in the life course.

A Note on Terms

Sufferers

I chose to call elders living with PD "Parkinson's disease sufferers" for several reasons. First, an acronym for the longer term "people living with Parkinson's disease," PWPD, seemed unwieldy and alienating. The medical term "Parkinson's patient" didn't seem to fit either, for as mentioned, PD sufferers don't really consider themselves to be sick. And while they often require medical care, I didn't want my reference to them to overemphasize that aspect of their lives. People with PD have been known to refer to themselves as "Parkinsonians," "PDs," and "Parkys," but the intimacy and sense of belonging attached to these terms made my use of them feel inappropriate. I chose to use the term "sufferer" to call attention to the numerous aspects of PD that work to produce suffering in their lives. "Suffering" is a term that forces a recognition of an individual's emotional, social, psychological, and physical experiences. It is imbued with negativity and pathos. In using it I both draw on the colloquial expression of the term "sufferer" to denote someone who is in the process of living with a burdensome physical, spiritual, or social condition, and acknowledge the moving and influential work of anthropologists who have explored the creation and reproduction of suffering within and between societies (Black and Rubinstein 2004; Kleinman, Das, and Lock 1996).

Older Adults and Elders

In the United States, old age is marked by retirement from the workforce, disability, menopause, the birth of grandchildren, the loss of a spouse, the beginning of pension or Social Security payments, or attaining a particular chronological age. These role transitions are accompanied by new terms denoting one's social status, such as "retiree," "widower," or "grandfather." There also exist a number of roleless terms with which to refer to adults nearing the end of the life course: Should we call them "senior citizens," "elders," "older adults," "sixty-five plus," "the aged," or "mature adults"? Each term carries a particular cultural tone, some negative and others neutral or positive. Throughout the book I choose to use the terms "elders" and "older adults" interchangeably. I recognize that the term "older adult" implies an implicit measurement against some undefined group of "younger adults" (connoting older adults' lesser value), and that "elder" is sometimes read as frail. Despite these negative casts, the book's focus on aging as a social process makes the term "older adults" an appropriate marker of difference making. Within anthropological discourse, the term "elder" denotes persons who have reached a knowledgeable social position from which to speak, which is invariably the case for those generous people whose experiences inform this book.

Caregivers

I use the term "caregiver" conscious of its implications. The term can imply a one-way provision of services to a dependent person, has a benevolent flavor, and can mask the intense physicality often involved with the role. Other terms, such as "carework," emphasize the demands of this role and remind us that such labors are often unpaid. "Bed and body work," a term used most often in long-term care literature, denotes the labor involved but, like "carework," implies that such activities are obligatory and deemphasizes their emotional and spiritual aspects. Among study participants there was a lack of consensus regarding terminology. Some caregivers explained that they couldn't be "caregivers" because they didn't provide enough help, while others demurred that such activities were a natural part of married life. Husbands and wives are by definition caregivers for each other. However, spouses living with quite disabled partners strongly claimed the term "caregiver," noting that activities like toileting or lifting their spouse were not normal aspects of married life. Adopting the role of caregiver helped them to preserve their marital relationship by cordoning off the activities deemed extramarital. My use of the term "caregiver" recognizes the social power of the term for some spouses and signals the uneasiness with which the role is adopted and maintained.

Plan of the Book

I introduce each chapter of the book with a narrative account taken from my field notes and interview transcripts to set the tone for the chapter and to introduce particular study participants, issues, or examples. Some of the stories conveyed in these narrative passages are humorous, and others saddening or shocking. I took special care to choose what I feel are representative examples and cases. As disturbing as some of the experiences are, be reminded that few of the stories in this book are of extreme or extraordinary cases. I have changed all the personal names and many of the place names to protect confidentiality. I have sometimes combined descriptions of support group conversations, events, and occasionally individual people to further conceal participants' identity.

Chapters 1 and 2 provide the theoretical and methodological framework for the study, as well as an overview of the biomedical understanding of PD. Chapters 3 through 7 each approach PD sufferers' experiences from a different aspect of an EM and work to briefly elucidate (1) the ways in which PD functions as a condition between illness and disease, and (2) how the embodiment of aging in the context of this condition is linked to sufferers' chronological age. Chapter 3 discusses the often-lengthy process of arriving at a PD diagnosis, and chapter 4 describes biomedical and sufferer-held definitions of PD. Chapter 5 presents sufferers' models for PD causation and highlights how PD is differentiated from normal aging. Chapter 6 explains the state of therapeutic interventions available at the time of my study and how sufferers' experience of seeking relief impacts their sense of growing older and living with a condition. Chapter 7 explores disease progression, how sufferers attribute blame to new somatic phenomena, and how blame plays into retirement decisions. Chapter 8 presents a dialogic discussion of caregiving and touches upon how the act of caregiving shapes the embodiment of aging for both giver and receiver. The concluding chapter discusses modes of embodiment in the case of PD and why we should consider PD and other chronic sicknesses *conditions*. There are two appendices: Appendix A contains brief descriptions of the sufferers whose words appear in this book, listed alphabetically by first name (pseudonym); appendix B provides a list of advocacy and other PD-related resources to assist persons looking for a PD community or other support.

2

Ethnography and Age in the Field

Introduction: Are You Working on a Cure?

The directions that Everett gave me over the phone took me out along the interstate, past thigh-high cornstalks and deep green fields of soybeans, and then along the meandering country highway that led into town. Even though I had lived in Iowa for a few years, to my mind "town" still connoted high-rise apartment buildings, traffic, and crowds. In Iowa, "town" can refer to a village of five hundred or to a small city of sixty thousand. Town, as opposed to "country," is where you go to shop, see the doctor, or perhaps attend church services. Country is where you live, independent and self-sufficient, for as long as you can manage. In the country, you take care of your own and you get by with what you have. When the time comes that you cannot manage the responsibilities country demands or when your neighbor's help can no longer fill the gap between what you can do for yourself and what needs to be done, then you move to town. Town living can have its problems, but it is often easier on one's body and pride to find a small house or apartment and live closer to the bank, post office, and doctors than to consider bringing in outside help—be it a visiting nurse or a nursing home.

As I crawled my way through a town of about twenty thousand, I wondered what to expect from a PD support group. I imagined the meeting to be a combination of an Alcoholics Anonymous meeting and an after-church fellowship coffee. But, despite (or perhaps due to) my extensive study of the PD literature, I had questions about the topic at hand—aging and Parkinson's—and about what fieldwork with PD sufferers would be like. How disabled might these people be? Would I be able to understand them? Would they be interested in my research, and would they be able to understand me? And, as a university person and a non-Iowa native, would my outsider status be insurmountable? These anxieties and questions are typical of any anthropologist setting out into the field for the first time, yet here I was just an hour or two from home. I was neither a "halfie," being a young and healthy outsider (Narayan 1993), nor "studying up" (Nader 1972)—that is, examining the hierarchies of power—nor enmeshing myself in the daily life of a small community. I wasn't traveling to some far-off locale; in fact, I was heading toward a destination we all have in common—old age. And, like many others, despite my planning and preparation I was unsure of what it had to offer.

I eased my foreign-made car with out-of-county plates into a spot between a dilapidated domestically made pickup truck and a large sedan. I was reminded of my fieldwork in rural Oklahoma, where my car always seemed to stand out among a sea of pickup trucks. I had parked a couple of blocks away to give myself a few moments to gather my thoughts, and as I now commonly do, to allow persons who really needed them the opportunity to park in the spots close to the building. The town had a small but lively business district nestled around a traditional town square and flanked by a few large manufacturing plants. The sidewalks were wide and unbroken, and traffic lights were infrequent.

I made my way to the building, consent forms, pens, and notebook in hand, and walked past a few older couples talking in the lobby. One woman was visibly shaking, her head nodding uncontrollably and her speech wavering. A younger man, perhaps in his fifties, was seated in a motorized chair trying to talk with an older gentleman. The younger one could barely speak; the older one could barely hear. I was in the right place. I nodded politely as I passed and made my way into the small meeting room. Everett stood up, introduced himself, and shook my hand. "Glad you could make it." He was taller than I had imagined and seemed strong, from his handshake. I knew that he suffered from a progressive and debilitating disease, but upon first glance Everett appeared to be a textbook example of successful aging. Regardless of my months of preparation, I consider this meeting to mark the beginning of my PD education.

A dozen or so group members slowly entered the room and found their seats, taking a few moments to visit with a friend, hang up their hats and coats (even though it was in the upper eighties), and adjust the window shades to reduce the brightness of the incoming light. Everett welcomed everyone back to their monthly meeting and asked them to introduce themselves, going around the circle. Other than the low hum of the air conditioner (making the room too cold for them and too warm for me), the room was rather quiet. I took in the drawn and somber expressions facing me and wondered, "What have I gotten myself into?" But as each person gave their name and offered a few comments on how long they had had PD and what kinds of symptoms they had, my interpretation of their expressions changed. I could see the slight intimation of a smile and hear the humor in their voices. I recognized that what I had taken for gravity in their expressions was really a symptom of the disorder, of what one man I later interviewed called "the mask." I had not realized that this fieldwork in my native country would present a challenge common to anthropological fieldwork—the misinterpretation of body language and hand signs. I would have to learn to look beyond facial expression and shaking hands to see a speaker's true meaning and intent, a social skill that was both difficult to acquire and challenging to practice.

When the introductions concluded, Everett welcomed me warmly with a few explanatory remarks: I was an anthropologist studying PD, and I was there to tell them about it for the day's program. When I had spoken with Everett about coming to the meeting, I had asked him for ten or fifteen minutes of their usual meeting time. I hadn't planned on being the main attraction. I stood up from my place in the circle and thanked the group for giving me the opportunity to speak with them. I explained that I was an anthropologist conducting research on PD and aging. I was not looking for a cure or the cause of PD; rather I wanted to hear from them how it had affected their lives. I shared with them a few of my questions: What were their first symptoms? Had they thought that these were signs of something serious? How long did it take them to get diagnosed? Had PD changed their retirement plans?

I told them that I had come to see if anyone would be interested in participating in my project. I hoped to attend their support group meetings as often as I could to observe and to participate to whatever degree they would like. Individuals would be asked to complete a questionnaire by mail and perhaps to let me come by with my tape recorder for an interview. I could not pay them anything, but I intimated that baked goods would serve as a consolation prize. I passed around participation forms and pens and waited for questions. The room was quiet. For a moment I feared that they could not hear my soft speaking voice well enough to take in everything that I had just shared (a challenge that I would face numerous times throughout the fifteen months of field research). Finally, the group came to life, proffering questions.

"Do you know anything about PSP?"

"Are you working on a cure?"

"I have been taking carbidopa-levodopa for six months and I cannot tell any difference. Do you think I should just stop taking it?"

Slowly, as I answered each question as best as I could, I was drawn into the circle. Our conversation turned away from my research to members' very specific questions about PD research, their personal medical history, medications, and resources. And then Rose spoke. Rose is a petite woman with PD, a back disfigured by osteoporosis-related kyphosis, madly shaking restless legs, and a warm sense of humor. She turned to me and asked, "Where did you say you were from?" Disarmed and relieved, I returned her smile and replied that I had been raised "back East." The conversation and questions reached out toward me to learn more about where I had lived, my family and my hobbies, the weather, and what route I had taken to get there that day. Participation forms were filled out and the project slowly began. "Yes, of course we will help you," the group seemed to be saying. "Just sit down a while and have some cookies and juice and we will get to that." It seemed that, as we do with old age, I had arrived at my destination before I realized it, and the tools I had brought and the preparations I had made were all good and fine but were of little value without a bite to eat and someone to share it with.

Anthropological Research in the Fields of Opportunity

Parkinson's and aging research both present complex sampling issues. How does one find research participants who may be so disabled that they rarely leave home or whose disease status is not monitored by any public health surveillance system? (PD activists, using similar strategies to Alzheimer's disease advocates, are working to establish national patient registries.) In a study on aging, how does one decide what constitutes "old"? Should a study of PD among older adults limit eligibility to adults who were diagnosed in later life or those who aged with PD from middle to later adulthood, or include both? These questions posed practical and epistemological matters for the project at hand.

As described in chapter 1, persons living with idiopathic PD are generally diagnosed on the identification of three of the four cardinal signs—bradykinesia (slowed movement), resting tremor, rigidity, and postural instability (a propensity to fall). Diagnosis is further confirmed when sufferers demonstrate a positive response to carbidopa-levodopa, the mainstay drug of PD treatment. Despite these seemingly clear diagnostic parameters, each case of PD can look remarkably different. One person in their forties may experience a mild resting tremor that progresses so slowly that they do not consider it a nuisance in need of treatment and diagnosis for decades. Another person may begin to have episodes of extreme tiredness, falls, and slowness in their eighties and consider these to be signs of normal aging. Or, fulfilling the statistical odds, a man in his midsixties may start to notice that his arm is stiff, that he has a slight tremor in one hand, that he seems to stumble more frequently, and that he has trouble picking up his feet to walk. Thus, while PD is certainly a diagnosable and widely recognized disorder, it also produces a notable degree of heterogeneity and is but one kind of parkinsonism (Rodnitzsky 2000). This diversity of disease presentation, course, and response to treatment has prompted some PD researchers to rethink the categorization of PD and to devise new models for understanding PD as a complex or constellation of related disorders (I discuss this in chapter 4).

In light of the variability in disease severity and presentation, I chose to invite participation from adults at least sixty years old who had a self-reported diagnosis of idiopathic PD, who maintained community residence, and who could communicate by speech in English. I selected the age of sixty as a lower cut-off because PD incidence increases with age, beginning at around sixty years old. Additionally, many Americans in this age cohort plan to retire at age sixty-five when they are eligible to receive Medicare and full Social Security benefits. By setting the minimum age at sixty I was able to include not only retirees, but also people who were planning their retirement, who managed careers with a chronic disorder, and who had to contend with workplace insurance coverage constraints. I elected to limit my sample to idiopathic PD sufferers to attain some level of homogeneity in somatic and illness experience. While PD differs widely from case to case, other forms of parkinsonism involve varying pharmacological interventions, prognoses, and symptoms. Idiopathic PD is likely the most common, treatable, and clearly defined variant of this constellation.

I opted to work exclusively with community-dwelling elders in order to obtain a sample that was as representative of the larger older adult population as possible. The majority of all older adults live in a private residence into late life, despite any disabilities. PD progression often causes considerable impairments, and some older PD sufferers do eventually seek community-based or long-term care. By working with community-dwelling PD patients I was able to gather information regarding challenges to their independence and aging in place. Over the course of the research, about two dozen of the study participants relocated to an assisted-living facility or nursing home or passed away. I had imagined that PD sufferers with severe speech deficits would self-select out of the interview portion of the study, yet in the end I conducted several interviews with persons who could barely speak. Finally, there were a number of reasons for conducting this study in Iowa. Iowa, being a predominantly agricultural state, demonstrates the challenges of aging with chronic illness in a rural area with its various geographic, economic, and cultural barriers to health care utilization. Iowa ranks among the top five states for PD prevalence (Lieberman 2002), and approximately 19 percent of Iowa's population is over sixty (U.S. Census Bureau 2000a). Given a modest prevalence rate of 1 percent among adults over sixty years old, in a state with an overall population just shy of three million people, 435,657 of them aged sixty-five or older, at least 4,300 PD sufferers reside in Iowa (FEDSTATS 2008). My work with roughly 200 of them represents around 4 percent of the affected population.

Locating Elder PD Sufferers

Given the range of physiological, cultural, and social variables involved in selecting an appropriate sample, most studies draw their PD participants from clinic populations or Medicare claims-based datasets (Rubenstein, Chrischilles, and Voelker 1997). These methods are biased in different ways. Clinic-based samples may be biased toward subjects positioned at either end of the economic continuum, the very poor or very wealthy. I was also wary of aligning myself too closely with medical providers, to avoid representing myself as a medical researcher and to avoid participating in the almost territorial turf battles over cultures of PD care. Medicare claims–based samples must rely on complicated means of assessing diagnosis. Because PD is not uniformly tracked or reported, subjects identified through this method would need to be defined as patients having had a clinic visit or hospitalization related to and coded for their PD during a specific period of time. Medicare claims data are heavily protected, expensive, and difficult to obtain. In light of these constraints, I chose to use a community-based snowball sample, inviting participation from PD support groups and through print advertisements in PD advocacy publications and regional newspapers.

Because PD does not express itself evenly across the landscape and because the population of some Iowa counties is "older" than others, I took out my Iowa roadmap, hung it on the wall, and drew a circle to represent my study area, which covered a two-hundred-mile radius centered on Iowa City—home of the state's tertiary care center and a prominent movement disorders clinic (see figure 1). This area not only represents a realistic driving distance from the center (with the farthest place being about a four-hour drive away), but also contains the full spectrum of rural and urban counties. It includes Iowa's most urban county (Polk, population 379,029) and smaller rural counties such as Washington (population 20,857) (U.S. Census Bureau 2004).

An Aging Heartland

In the American popular imagination, Iowa, centrally located in the heartland, is a homogenous landscape of religiously and politically conservative, friendly, family-oriented farmers living in rambling picturesque houses scattered among cornfields or clustered in quaint insular towns. While Iowa's industrialized factory farms, illegal methamphetamine production, or state-of-the-art neurosurgery usually do not constitute the imagined Iowa, to some extent the stereotypes ring true. Iowa is a rural state with a population of less than three million (U.S. Census Bureau 2004). Des Moines, the most heavily urbanized area, is home to about 200,000 Iowans. Most Iowans live in small towns averaging fewer than 10,000 persons. Surrounding these towns are the vast soybean and cornfields that give Iowa its characteristic rolling, expansive landscape. About 89 percent of Iowa's land is in farms, and Iowa ranks first in the nation for the production of corn, eggs, and pork (IDALS 2006). Many people may understand that farm life is not a relaxed idyllic existence, but the nature of farming and rural life has undergone dramatic changes over the past fifty years. In 1950s Iowa, there were over 34.4 million acres of farmland in production; in 2004 this area had decreased by 2.5 million acres. Not only are fewer people farming in Iowa, they are doing so on larger farms (IDALS 2006). Almost all who participated in this project lived in a rural area at some point in their life. Those elders who continued to reside in the country still commonly lived in farmhouses, but only a handful still actively farmed the land.

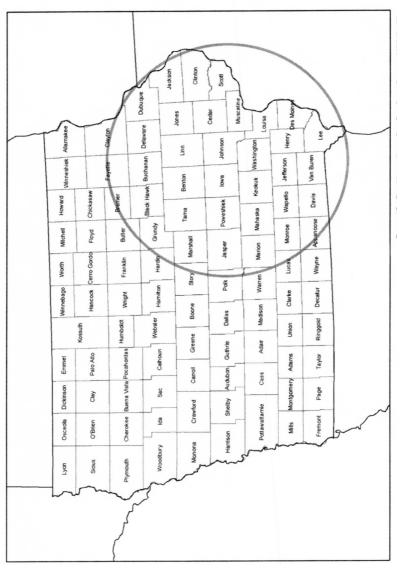

Prepared By: State Library of Iowa, State Data Center Program, 800-248-4483,
http://www.iowadatacenter.org

FIGURE 1 Study area: the state of Iowa and its counties

Land use and demography are changing in Iowa, but many older Iowans preserve their ties to the homeplace. Having leased their land to family or other community members, they remained in their homes and planned to do so for as long as they could manage. Iowans age in place. About one-fifth of elder Iowans reside in one of the five major cities. More than three-quarters of Iowans over the age of sixty-five were born in the state and only 7.5 percent reside in a nursing home (IDEA 2006). This lack of mobility and the outflow of younger Iowans makes Iowa an aging state, with more than 7 percent of its population over the age of seventy (U.S. Census Bureau 2004).

Across the United States, rural states such as Iowa are home to the largest proportion of elders (McLaughlin and Jensen 1998). Compared to urban dwellers, rural people have lower socioeconomic status, more chronic health conditions, less access to and acceptance of formal health care services, and more transportation barriers (Shenk 1998). Rural elders have higher rates of disability than their urban counterparts, and they have lower incomes, less education, and poorer housing (Kelley and MacLean 1997; Krout 1994, 1997; Krout and Coward 1998; Mockenhaupt and Muchow 1994; Redford and Severns 1994). In 2000, about 38 percent of Iowans aged sixty-five and older lived with at least one disability, and about 7 percent of Iowa seniors lived below the poverty line (U.S. Census Bureau 2000b). About half of America's rural elders are married (McLaughlin and Jensen 1998). Those who cannot rely upon a spouse for day-to-day assistance are presented with a small pool of able or available community members because fewer working-age adults reside in rural areas (Parker et al. 1992). "Thus, living arrangement and marital status can combine with small community size to place elders in a more vulnerable position with respect to access to formal services and to the availability of networks of informal services" (McLaughlin and Jensen 1998, 39). Rural elders who live alone are likely to reside in homes in need of maintenance and upkeep to maintain safety and independence, but are unlikely to possess the financial or social resources to avoid having to relocate to a care facility in later life (Krout 1994).

This social and political economic climate poses challenges for those who live with a chronic illness such as PD and illustrates the special barriers facing elders who live in rural and semirural areas. PD sufferers often require long-term care, costly prescription medications, a wide range of ancillary services, home health visits, and numerous physician visits and phone calls (Chrischilles et al. 1998; Fischer 1999; Rubenstein, Chrischilles, and Voelker 1997). Accompanying these needs are increased economic burdens that are often out-of-pocket and that arise in periods of unemployment or retirement when income may be fixed or limited (Fitzsimmons and Bunting 1993; Rubenstein, DeLeo, and Chrischilles 2001). The limitations of rural medical practice stem from the small population base and providers' desire for individual autonomy and authority (Shortell et al. 2000). While at times this means that rural dwellers receive all their care from general practitioners and rarely consult specialists, it also means that patients often are able to build meaningful and longstanding relationships with their physicians. However, the three national PD advocacy organizations recommend that patients seek treatment from neurologists specializing in movement disorders.

Iowa City is at the heart of complex care coordination for a majority of older Iowans and is located at the center of the project's study area. Iowans living south or north of the study area may travel to either Illinois or to Iowa City for their care. A majority of the PD sufferers in this study had been to the movement disorders clinic at the University of Iowa (UI) in Iowa City at some point in their PD career. Iowans residing in the extreme western part of the state generally travel farther west to Nebraska for care. A few people in the northern and northeastern part of the study area travel up to the Mayo Clinic in Rochester, Minnesota, or to Milwaukee, Wisconsin, for care. And, as I will discuss in later chapters, even within the heart of this region a number of people traveled more than four hours one way to see a specific neurologist whom they perceived to be especially skilled in treating PD. In addition to the UI clinics, Iowa PD patients can receive specialized PD care at a number of locations: at Veteran's Health Administration hospitals, from neurologists who travel to the smaller hospitals, at medium-sized regional hospitals such as the ones in Cedar Falls or Burlington, or at the PD clinic in Des Moines.

Generally speaking, Iowans have access to a diverse assortment of adjunctive therapies. They can visit practitioners at a college of osteology, more than six different schools of therapeutic massage, Maharishi Ayurved University, Palmer School of Chiropractic (Iowa is the birthplace of chiropractic), or privately operating providers of acupuncture, herbology, homeopathy, Reiki, reflexology, or naturopathy. Such modalities are often termed "complementary and alternative," but in the case of PD they are squarely adjunctive. PD sufferers may use such therapies in addition to seeing a neurologist or general practitioner, but I never encountered any older PD sufferers who used them in place of biomedical treatment.

I identified eligible participants through formal presentations at PD support group meetings, announcements in PD advocacy publications, paid announcements in regional newspapers, and by word of mouth. I worked with thirteen PD support groups in the study area. A majority are grass-roots affairs, having taken shape when a newly diagnosed patient felt the need for a support community. Several groups were sponsored by area hospitals and were facilitated by hospital staff. Crossing both models were eight that were connected to a larger advocacy network. I contacted the support group facilitators and gained permission to attend a regularly scheduled monthly meeting to present a description of my research and invite participation. All these groups expressed interest in the project and assisted in varying degrees with my recruitment efforts.

Doing Ethnography and Participant Observation

Traditional anthropological research involves ethnographic observation within the confines of a culturally and often geographically bounded community. Yet this discursive tradition has been challenged by feminist and medical anthropologists seeking to understand both broad political-economic forces as well as the microcultures created by various sickness communities. The prevalence and experience of sickness can be endemic or diffuse within a particular population. In the case of PD, while it is a relatively common neurological disorder for adults over the age of sixty, it is an uncommon condition when viewed across the entire age distribution of any one community. The stigmatization of PD sufferers intensifies the challenge of defining a community for study. Older PD sufferers are less likely to have opportunities to meaningfully engage with the larger community and commonly report feeling embarrassed by their symptoms in public (Nijhof 1995; Strauss and Corbin 1984). Thus, I sought PD sufferers from the area around a central, culturally significant location to participate in the study.

With this choice, my study "follows the disease" and engages a popular sampling approach in medical anthropology and ethnography (Marcus 1998; Martin 1997). By allowing the disease to stand in as a proxy for community and locating PD throughout eastern Iowa, I was able to generate flexibility in defining a study population and community. This approach also supported my desire to minimize the marginalization of an already stigmatized group by focusing on PD sufferers as subjects rather than as "people with a disease" (Whyte and Ingstad 1995). This multisited research allowed me to widen my scope from my preconceived notions of important cultural variables to a sufferer-defined set of salient ideas, experiences, and social structural institutions. Marcus's ideas about multisited ethnography, which gained notoriety within anthropological circles a decade ago, bear repeating here, as they not only reinforce the value of such an ethnographic project but also remind us of the weight of disciplinary tradition: "Thus, in multi-sited ethnography, comparison emerges from putting questions to an emergent object of study whose contours, sites and relationships are not known beforehand, but are themselves a contribution of making an account that has different, complexly connected real-world sites of investigation" (1998, 86). That following the disease and multisited ethnography still feel like new and revolutionary ways of doing ethnography speaks more to the entrenchment of culture within geography than it does to the novelty of this trend in medical anthropological research.

Yet, even in industrialized nations such as the United States, there remains a connection to the landscape, especially in predominantly rural places such as Iowa. Here, instead of life revolving around the happenings in town, town seems to reflect the happenings of life at home, on the farm or in the country. So while I endeavored to follow PD wherever it occurred in eastern Iowa, I was also at once compelled to situate its experience within the local and regional goings on. Time grounded this sometimes contradictory method. Participant observation normally implies a lengthy, intensive engagement as a nominally accepted member of a community. Participant observation can be done quickly, as those who use rapid ethnographic assessment methods know, but such speedy work is almost always seen as a method of last resort. The temporal aspect of fieldwork meshed well with my research topic, as both aging and PD occur over long periods of time. It is rare to see aging happening moment by moment, or in the span of a day or week. And, while PD progression and its unpredictability can produce remarkable change from one day to the next, it is the norm within the heterogeneity that impairments and progression are marked month by month, year by year—from Christmas dinner to Christmas dinner or from one year's annual physical to the next.

Cultural anthropologists strive to achieve a location of intersubjectivity, a socially contentious role, between participant and observer (Tedlock 1991). This position creates an epistemological and social tension that drives research questions, builds rapport with study participants, and produces ethical and personal quandaries for which there are few straightforward or right responses. Participant observation for this study took place during support group meetings, in patient education seminars and conferences, and in participants' homes during interviews and visits. The PD support groups generally met monthly, and by the end of the study period I had attended more than one hundred meetings. My participation during such meetings varied from group to group. Some of the groups were formal affairs led by hospital staff and allowed little space for questions or interpersonal interaction. I always arrived early for these meetings, as did a number of PD sufferers and their spouses, to have time to get to know people and for them to get to know me. The PD sufferer-facilitated groups functioned more as support systems, with attendees sharing their ideas and experiences with each other in the hope of learning something new and helping others feel more normal. My participation in these groups depended a bit on the day's topic. One day I might be asked to chime in with my opinion on a recent study or PD-related news item, while on another I was more or less relegated to the background as people hashed out their frustrations and shared their joys.

As an observer, always, I was taking notes. My field notes detail support group discussion topics and how they were received, friendly gossip pertaining to other group members, literature distributed during meetings, and observations describing the month-to-month changes in participants' lives. Such observation notes are an important counterpoint to the other kinds of data that I went on to collect. Support group observations seemed to provide a snapshot of people's best efforts. These groups functioned as safe spaces for physical "deviance"— social places where it was perfectly acceptable to drool, shake, spill your juice, use a cane, or express irritation with medications or doctors. At the same time, these meetings were also social events attended by people with whom you might have gone to high school, conducted business, or attended church. While everyone I encountered certainly respected others' privacy, the appearance of successful coping and slow progression was important to many attendees. You could "let it all hang out" at a support group meeting, but some people took pains to downplay the severity of their symptoms, financial problems, or caregiving burdens. There are two universals among Iowan PD sufferers: No one wants to be viewed as someone to be pitied by others, and no one wants to be thought of as someone who complains or is ungrateful for what they have.

How does an able-bodied, thirty-something, nonnative Iowan participate in the world of rural Iowan PD sufferers? My involvement in life outside support group meetings consisted of providing an informal information and referral service and acting as a dinner guest, family friend, and confidante. When I set out to conduct this study I imagined that my age would present the greatest barrier to research. My younger age did lead some people to relate to me as a grandchild-at-large, but on the whole, once I had formed a relationship with someone, as Fry points out, "the age just disappeared" (2006). What did create social distance was my university affiliation, and to a lesser extent, the fact that I was not born in Iowa. Generally speaking, I was incorporated into the support group setting and people's individual lives as a "university person" to whom they could direct questions and speak with confidentiality. I understood this clearly when one older man asked me, "What did you say you were called again? Anthropologist? I had to tell the fellas at the coffee shop that I couldn't come by today. Next time I see them, I can tell them that I was seeing my anthropologist."

Knowing a university person and taking part in research gave some people bragging rights, but a few others viewed me with suspicion. One woman wrote on her questionnaire: "All of this PD research on the news never seems to reach me." This frustration with the lack of translational research and real progress in PD treatment was rarely directed toward me, but it arose often enough that I frequently questioned both my research motivations and my standard for success. Anthropologists have long grappled with the issue of whether the human connections forged via ethnography require us to identify real-world applications for our findings or if having a political or humanistic agenda might sully the theoretical rigor of one's research. I struggled to make clear to PD sufferers and their families that my goal was to improve the understanding of aging with a condition such as PD, and that, while I hoped that improved care would arise from this understanding, I could not promise it. This goal was accepted at face value, though at times I recognized that it might ring hollow in the face of the suffering that I witnessed.

The pace of fieldwork among older adults, and perhaps especially in rural areas, is slow. Early on in the research, a colleague of mine and I shared notes on our day. She was conducting research on the film production process and insider/outsider status in Hollywood (see Ono 2001). She once arrived at a coffee shop for an interview to find that it was valet parking only, the lot was full, and the interviewee had allotted just a few minutes to speak with her. It could take her an hour to drive 15 miles. In comparison, I drove 140 miles along rural highways in about two hours to meet with someone for three hours over bottomless cups of decaffeinated coffee. Where she had to attend black tie affairs in three-inch high heels and makeup, I found myself dressing in modest, conservative clothing. My informants had to cut interviews short to take medications or naps. Her informants interrupted "face time" to answer phone calls, to order martinis, or to run off to another engagement.

A brief passage describing a typical day in the field (adapted from my field notes) is illustrative.

When I got up this morning it was already in the upper eighties and the sun's brightness felt unrelenting. It would be another day where I had to carry my equipment with me wherever I went, lest my cassette tapes melt in the car. I gathered my overnight bag, tape recorder, notebooks, forms, and maps and started out for Windybluff. It usually takes me about two hours to get there, but with the weather forecasters warning of thirty-five-mile-per-hour winds I knew it would be longer. Windybluff is a medium-sized town for Iowa, located in the northeastern part of the state. There are no straight roads to get there, only a series of curving two-lane highways that take you past small dairy farms, soybean fields, and sometimes, it seemed, a whole lot of nothing.

I arrived in the early afternoon between lunch and nap time, just as the support group meeting was getting started. A few people recognized me from the last time and I noticed both some missing faces and others that were new to me. The facilitator announced the topic for the day's meeting, "Tips for Managing Common Complaints," and started an informal conversation on ways to decrease drooling, to avoid falls, and to maximize the benefit of carbidopa-levodopa through carefully timed protein intake. The group discussed this for a bit and then the organized conversation devolved into smaller chats between old friends and the newcomers.

The man sitting next to me asked me how my research was going and I gave him a rundown on how many people had enrolled and what kinds of things I had been up to. He explained to me that his "biggest gripe" was that no two doctors seemed to have the same diagnosis. He went to one doctor who told him that he had essential tremor. Months later he saw a different physician who diagnosed him with PD. A few years ago he decided to have deep brain stimulation (DBS) surgery and now he needs to have the battery changed at a cost of $20,000. His insurance company does not want to pay for it because he has to go to an out-of-network hospital for the procedure. Making matters worse is the fact that he has to drive three hours each way to see his new PD doctor.

All around us people were having similar conversations about driving, doctors who can't seem to hear what their patients are saying (to my mind both literally and figuratively), and the high cost of medications. The woman seated on my other side spoke to me about her recent struggle with public restrooms. "I just don't know how I can keep doing this." She described how difficult it was for her to manage her husband's toileting in public spaces. He needed her assistance to undress and navigate the restroom stall. She asked me, "Should I be bringing him into the women's restroom or should I keep trying to use the men's with him? I just can't stay home all of the time and I can't leave him at home alone, either." We talked a bit about strategies that she could use to ensure their privacy and protect her husband's dignity in such situations, but it seemed that she was less interested in devising solutions than she was in just having someone to talk to who understood where she was coming from without a lengthy explanation. As interested as I was to learn more about her experience, I had mixed feelings about the way in which she treated her spouse. Throughout our discussion she constantly referred to him as a problem, which in itself was not troublesome, but she did so while he was seated next to her. While I could not be sure that he heard her (her constantly having to shout to be heard was another issue), I felt badly for him as I empathized with her. A common feeling these days.

After the snack of juice and store-bought cookies the meeting disbanded and we said our goodbyes. It was late afternoon and so I headed over to a local hotel to check in and drop off my bags before having dinner at the home of a couple who lived in town. The next day I had both morning and afternoon interviews scheduled. At nine A.M. I would be driving forty miles north to meet with a couple out on their dairy farm for a few hours, then I would drive back down through town for lunch before an afternoon interview appointment with a couple who lived right off of the main square. Around dinner time I would then head back out on the road toward my home, to think through what I had learned, to transcribe interviews, eke out some field notes, and prepare for the next trip, in three days' time.

Counting on the Data: Quantitative Tools

Cultural anthropology is characterized primarily as a qualitative discipline, but quantitative data are almost always collected as a part of ethnographic research. Thus, even though the ethnographic project focuses heavily upon fieldwork and the narratives it produces, anthropologists recognize that "science cannot be spoken in a singular universal voice. Any methodological standpoint is, by definition, partial, incomplete, and historically contingent. Diversity of representations is needed" (Riessman 1993, 70). The questionnaire and field notes data provide such diversity. Field notes produce highly detailed, nuanced descriptions of individual conversations, observations, and interactions. Questionnaires, by contrast, gather depersonalized data in preestablished categories from a large number of people. The nearsightedness of field notes is balanced by the farsightedness of questionnaires, or in another discourse, field notes speak about individuals and questionnaires tell us about populations.

I designed and pilot-tested two questionnaires—one which was sent to caregivers and one which was designed for PD sufferers—to assist me with the collection and organization of countable information. This included items as varied as: educational attainment; birth year; employment status and history; marital status; symptom frequency; out-of-pocket medication expenses and insurance support; driving distances to physicians; comorbidities, falls, and unintentional injuries; year diagnosed and type of provider diagnosing; health care utilization in the prior twelve months; use of community-based, in-home services such as an emergency call button or respite care; self-assessed need for assistance with a list of home-related tasks; PD-related medications; use of complementary, adjunctive, and surgical therapies; participation in clinical trials; driving status; markers of social engagements such as volunteer or faith community activities; PD support group attendance; and hobbies or leisure activities. Drawing upon my public health training, I included the RAND 36-Item Health Survey 1.0 (also known as the Medical Outcomes Survey [MOS]) (RAND Corporation 2006; Ware 1993). The RAND MOS is a standardized measurement of reported health status that can help illustrate the efficacy of current therapies or indicate future intervention areas (Chrischilles et al. 1998; RAND Corporation 2006; Rubenstein, Chrischilles, and Voelker 1997; Ware 1995; Ware and Sherbourne 1992).

The questionnaire data contributed to two key goals. First, the questionnaires allowed me to collect population-level data from a larger sample of people than I would be able to get to know on a one-on-one basis over the course of a year. These data not only provided background information for selecting interview participants on the criteria of age and sex, but also allowed me to assess how representative of the larger group the interviewees were. Second, the questionnaires enabled me to establish a rough measure of disease severity against which I could compare any narrative themes or patterns. With that failsafe, I could have confidence that the narrative analysis holds together across multiple demographic and health-related variables. The caregiver questionnaires also contribute to two key components of the study. By collecting similar information from caregivers and PD sufferers, I was able to compare their reports of PD symptoms and assistance provided by spouses. And the open-ended items on the caregiver instrument emerged as a safe and confidential space for caregivers to voice their frustrations, disgust, and sorrow or to ask me questions.

Explanatory Models and Illness Narratives on the Ground

My observation notes were critical to contextualize support group and other interactions. However, from the initial planning stages onward, I knew that intensive, focused interviews would comprise the most powerful and rich data of the entire project. As I discussed in chapter 1, I integrated a structured mode of enquiry, the explanatory model (EM), with an unstructured method, the illness narrative. In this way I hoped that the interviews would (1) be comparable to each other, (2) demonstrate the heterogeneity inherent in PD sufferers' conceptions of the disorder, and (3) capture what PD sufferers believed to be the most life-altering aspects of this disordering experience. More than 100 caregivers and 148 PD sufferers volunteered to participate in interviews. Using questionnaire data, I sorted potential interviewees by current age and gender and set out to interview equal numbers of men and women (thirty-five each), distributed among the decades of life represented—sixth, seventh, and eighth. Over the course of nine months I conducted seventy-one interviews, ranging in length from forty-five minutes to more than two hours. In addition, I had planned to interview ten caregivers (five men and five women) whose partners were too disabled to participate. Yet when I began the PD interviews I found that some participants strongly preferred to have their spouses present, and so I conducted thirty of the interviews with couples. I conducted three additional interviews with caregivers of severely impaired PD sufferers. I tape-recorded almost all the interviews (sixty-nine), and I conducted all but two in participants' homes.

Conducting the interviews was both an enjoyable and difficult experience, and not simply because of the subject matter's emotional weight. The informed consent process was occasionally alienating, but I value such mechanisms to protect research participants' rights and to serve as a reminder that as researchers we must be vigilant to maintain our identity as interested outsiders with preestablished goals and limitations. Tape recording, which I had thought might intimidate people, was universally accepted. Because PD can decrease speech volume and intelligibility, participants were reassured by lapel microphones that could capture their speech without their having to strain their voice to be heard. While microphones did help immensely during transcription, during the interviews I often found myself leaning in, trying to understand what the person seated two feet away was trying to tell me.

Interpersonal communication, as I alluded to in the introduction to this chapter, was an ongoing learning process. Some of PD and PD medications' effects on the body, such as:

Unexpected sleep episodes and somnolence

Dysarthria (difficulty in producing clear speech without a stutter)

Slowed cognitive function

Hand, arm, or leg tremor

Heightened emotionality

Anxiety and depression, or

Decreased facial affect

expressed themselves in interviews as:

Interviewees dozing off for a few moments in midsentence

Participants' speech becoming garbled, hoarse, slow, and unintelligible to me

Participants requiring long periods of time to consider and respond to questions, or being able to respond only to direct questions

Interviewees' hands, arms, or legs shaking, silent in person but creating loud tapping noises on the tape, obscuring the recorded conversation

A spontaneous argumentative or persecutory stance or unanticipated bouts of crying on the part of interviewees

Interviewees suddenly changing the topic to death and dying

Participants' difficult-to-interpret body language, such as squinting, head nodding, or hand gestures

But these challenges were not insurmountable, and I was repeatedly struck by the generosity and openness of the many people who volunteered to be in the study. Participants invited me into their homes to share with me their views on the indignities of aging, the frustrations of PD treatment, and the challenges of adapting to PD's symptoms. Caregivers wept at the changes in their partners and their sense of guilt during those moments of anger and resentment. Caregivers offered important historical vantage points on the illness experiences, filling gaps in information and presenting contrasting interpretations of meaning and the valuation of PD-related life changes. PD sufferers described their economic worries; embarrassment at their visible tremor or at falling in public spaces; their feelings of guilt at having burdened their spouse; the shame of sexual dysfunction, drooling, or memory impairment; and the ways in which they maintained their identity and dignity in the face of serious life changes. I came away from these encounters by turns bemused, depressed, anxious, or grief stricken. Occasionally, I felt endangered by participants' sexual advances, anxieties, or vivid hallucinations. There were also sporadic instances in which I explored my ethical responsibility to report possible spousal abuse, self-neglect, or unsafe drivers.

I was not able to compensate participants for their time, but I did little things consistent with local etiquette to express my appreciation and establish a minimal level of reciprocity. For example, I arrived for interviews with home-baked treats in hand, drove people to support group meetings, conducted library research for them and circulated relevant articles, and by request I shared inform-ation on community-based services, assisted-living options, case management, and falls and unintentional injury prevention. Every interview was followed up with a handwritten thank-you note and a typewritten transcript.

Finding Sense in the Data: Analysis and Management Techniques

Ethnography is by nature an analytical endeavor: Analysis is ongoing in the field, but more intensively conducted after the fieldwork has concluded. I jotted down all my field notes by hand and then fleshed them out in greater detail as electronic documents later in the day or upon my return from a trip. Interviews produced both handwritten observational notes and tape recordings. I expanded upon these notes as electronic files separately from the interview transcripts. I transcribed the interviews over several months. As alluded to earlier in this chapter, even with lapel microphones the tape recordings were difficult to com-prehend. It could require ten hours to transcribe two hours of tape. I shared the transcripts with participants to validate information, offer an opportunity for clarification, and stimulate further discussion of particular themes (Riessman 1993). I kept all files secure on my home computer. A password-protected per-sonal digital assistant proved indispensable in the field as a reference for driv-ing directions, contact information, and appointments.

Field notes, interview notes and transcripts, and responses to the open-ended items from the two questionnaires were imported into a qualitative soft-ware package, NVIVO 2.0. This software served as an important tool with which to mine the qualitative data. These files were coded, and the codes were organ-ized into hierarchical trees. Coding served as a complex and flexible indexing system for the data; codes can be renamed, recoded, coded within, moved, or deleted with ease. Once I established an overall coding framework, I examined relationships between particular codes and the attributes of individual docu-ments. As Richards summarizes: "The goal is that by maintaining on-line, within one project, different evolving documents; retaining analytic processes for reapplication as theories, results, and goals change; and shaping and reshaping the bodies of material that represent different ways of looking, researchers can draw hugely varied materials together, maintaining a whole that is complex but entirely accessible for synthesis" (1999, 424).

Multimethod research poses a challenge to traditional anthropological lit-erary forms. Often, quantitative data are awarded a separate and distinct sec-tion of the text, and many times they are limited to a few descriptive statistics (Chibnik 1985). The interplay of qualitative and quantitative information in this study warrants literary integration, as each kind of data served as confirmation and counterpoint to the other. I first coded narrative data by topic (e.g., driving, relocation, or the EM constructs) and then by theme (such as fear of falling or the overlap between PD progression and aging). I then grouped the themes together and refined and redefined them as their relationship to the overarching research questions became more apparent. The narrative data provide detailed examples of the changes to retirement plans, identity, and interpersonal relationships that PD requires. The quantitative data provided via the questionnaires allowed me to determine whether an individual's health-related quality of life, age, use of services, and PD symptoms had statistical bearing on the particular codes and themes in their narrative. I used a statistical software package to calculate the RAND MOS measures, following the methods outlined in Ware (1993) and RAND (2006). I then imported code data to create an integrated data set. By integrating data sets in this way, I am able to demonstrate how quantitative information can reinforce the interpretation of narrative, and to honor the heterogeneity of illness narratives by contextualizing them within a range of PD experiences and life in Iowa.

Participants

Approximately 300 people enrolled in the study. PD sufferers tended to be married (84 percent) and well educated (60 percent had attended a trade school or had a college degree). The average age of PD sufferers was 73.5 years (SD 8.16 years); they had been diagnosed with PD in their midsixties (mean 64.9, SD 9.0 years) and had lived with the disorder for an average of 8 years (SD 5.3). Of the 171 PD sufferers who enrolled in the study, 71 percent completed the questionnaire and 71 participated in an interview. Caregivers were slightly younger than PD sufferers, with an average age of 70 years (SD 9.96 years). Of the 188 caregivers in the project, 65 percent completed questionnaires and 30 participated in an interview. While I made efforts to work with a racially diverse sample, Iowa is 94 percent white (FEDSTATS 2008), and all enrollees were white.

Aging or PD?

The allocation of blame for somatic changes in later life speaks to underlying beliefs concerning normal aging. In numerous ways, PD is experienced as a condition that both reflects and reproduces the belief that the story of growing older is one of growing sicker. Sufferers' diagnostic trajectories were almost as varied as the individuals themselves, and while some of the narratives illustrate the premise that aging people and even physicians sometimes mistake PD symptoms for those of normal aging, there were as many stories of people who sought care as soon as their symptoms appeared. And to my surprise, age at onset bore little relationship to the length of time between symptoms onset and diagnosis. What I came to understand, in moving my focus from elders' discovery of their sickness to being sick, is that age is an important part of people's experience in living with PD but that chronological age acquired this meaning after a diagnosis was conferred. Virtually everyone believed that growing older would compel them to make compromises based on what their bodies and minds could still do, but very few were prepared for the sometimes drastic differences between the old age they had imagined and the aging with PD they now experienced. As chapters 3 through 8 show, PD figures as a condition that both arises in and changes the aging process.

3

It Takes a Little While
to Find Out for Sure

Introduction: I Was a Little Disappointed

Peter and Laura live in a modest apartment in the center of town, just off the main square. I met them on a sunny morning in early summer, when their window garden was just beginning to burgeon with tomatoes, lettuce, and herbs. Laura greeted me at the door and gave me a quick tour of their apartment. It was a small two-bedroom with a patio and eat-in kitchen. Their furniture seemed to dominate the rooms, a consequence of their having downsized from a large home. About five years earlier Peter and Laura were finding it increasingly difficult to keep up with the maintenance a "proper home" required. Meticulous, neat, and proud, they preferred to relocate rather than let their home fall into disrepair. While Peter explained to me that "we just decided to get out," Laura interjected, "It was getting harder for you to do the work outside. [Your PD] was really, I think, the main reason we moved."

We settled into our chairs at the kitchen table, soaking up the morning sun and enjoying some coffee, and turned our conversation to PD and how Peter came to know that he had it. At first he told me that he was diagnosed a year ago; then he corrected himself and said two years. Laura interrupted, prompting him a bit, and he explained, "Well, the only thing is I knew somebody that had PD, and I thought maybe I might be acting like him. But then, I really didn't know. Laura must have had an inkling ahead of time. . . . I had a problem of some kind and I thought maybe it was AD [Alzheimer's disease], something like that. But it didn't turn out that way. And then later on the doctor said that he thought it was PD."

I asked him: "Do you have memory problems? Is that why you thought it was Alzheimer's?" He smiled and gestured to his wife, "You don't remember [poorly] like I do. Yeah, I do have memory problems, terrible memory problems. Well, it seems as though I plan on doing something and I get up to do it and when I get there I can't remember what I was going to do." Laura added, "But also, Peter, when I bring up something that happened a couple of weeks ago then anymore you can't remember what that was until I start repeating everything and then it sort of comes to you. [You forget] some things, not everything. Right?" This exchange typified our meeting that morning, as Peter suffered from mild memory impairments and substantial cognitive slowing. Peter would make a comment, and Laura would prompt him, hinting at the rest of the story, easing him back into familiar shared memories of the past decade.

About eight years ago Peter's hands started shaking. The couple would be in church sharing a hymnal when Laura would feel the book begin to quiver. They went to Peter's physician, who had been treating him for a number of years, and asked him whether he thought it might be PD. The family doctor said he did not think so, but over several visits they continued to ask, "Could this be PD?" He neither diagnosed it as PD nor referred their concerns to a neurologist or other specialist. Laura expressed her frustration with him, saying, "I think he's one that wants to do it himself, you know. He's smart, to talk to, but he wants to be in control, I think." After four years of progressive tremor and weakness, the family doctor told Peter that he did indeed have PD. Laura sighed. "But I was a little disappointed that he [doctor] waited that long before he was convinced that it was Parkinson's."

Peter's shaking hands had progressed considerably since then. He had virtually no control over his right arm and possessed limited mobility in his left. Eating and drinking were embarrassingly difficult, but he still managed to drive his pickup—he traded in his standard for an automatic transmission to do so. That spring the progression seemed to have sped up, and Peter felt more and more impaired as the weeks passed. I asked him which symptoms troubled him the most. He had difficulty deciding—they all caused him great distress. He couldn't control his hands, suffered from a generalized loss of strength and stamina, and was beleaguered by memory problems, he said.

> I wish I could talk better. My ideas affect my speech. Yeah. I have a little trouble getting it together, what I want to say. . . . I'll tell you. I went to the ball game the other day in Des Moines. And we was coming out of the amphitheater and every time there was a step I couldn't hardly handle myself. I have to hold onto the seats or onto the side. And pretty soon there was a lady coming along and said, "Are you having trouble?" or something like that and she let me hold on to her. Well, I got to be more careful going down that I don't overstep the step or something, you know. And then you rock forward [and fall]. And you got to be a little bit careful with that.

Laura added, "He's so sleepy." Then, to Peter: "You have weakness, too. Weakness. You can't walk, you are so tired."

Peter continued to see his family doctor for his PD care and had never been to see a neurologist. He stopped midsentence to retrieve a medium-sized plastic bin stuffed with pill bottles of varying shapes and sizes, virtually all marked with a prescription label. "It's a wonder you can eat!" I said. Laura replied, dryly, "We've had a bill for what was it, seven thousand dollars [laughs] last year because we both are on so much medication." They do not carry a private prescription drug insurance plan, and Medicare Part D had not yet been implemented. Despite the volume and number of medicines Peter was taking, Laura commented that they did not seem to work. Peter countered, "If I take them regularly at the right time, it seems to help. I think it seems to help, some. No, well, I mean I feel better. Maybe I'm just proud of myself that I didn't forget them."

We spoke a bit about a typical day for Peter and the kinds of things that he enjoyed doing. He managed to take a daily walk over to the city park and back, a distance of about six blocks. He watched television, tended to his tomatoes, and enjoyed just spending time with Laura. And every day he climbed into his pickup truck to head uptown for coffee with a handful of other retired men. He had a great deal of trouble following the conversation, and by the time he could think of a reply to someone's comment, the conversation had often moved on. However, he continued to go for the camaraderie he shared with this eclectic and supportive bunch.

Peter defined PD in this way:

Well, I'd say I'm losing my ability to walk, losing my ability to think good, and I'm losing my ability to talk. I can't walk too good. It just is a downhill struggle. And the shaking. It is frustrating. It's getting to be more frustrating all of the time. I have trouble with buttons. [Laura helps me] quite a lot. Quite a lot. [I used to help her with the dishes.] I did for a while. But it gets to where—I think one of the most confusing things in the whole works is that your hands are [uncoordinated], just like your hands are tied. I want to put my shirt in my pants and I can't hardly get them to go where I want to. And it just frustrates you. Like to get a handkerchief out of my pocket. I can get the handkerchief out and want to blow my nose, but I can't hardly get my handkerchief shaped in a way that I can handle it. [If you are at a store and] you break a twenty-dollar bill and you've got five ones or something like that and you try to get them back in there and you just can't hardly make it go.

There was a while if I got real busy I would improve enough that I could handle [myself] almost. It is not perfect, but it makes a lot of difference. But anymore I can't get enough exercise, I guess. But I get trouble with my hearing aids, too. And when I get coffee, I don't hear the other guys. I can't understand them, in a way. I don't know whether that has anything to do with Parkinson's or not.

Laura interrupted Peter to make some consoling comments. He helps her as he can, she assured him. She doted on her husband, and the only tension between the two seemed to be Peter's hearing loss, perhaps the most common cause of marital arguments I heard over the course of the project. Peter either forgot to put his hearing appliances in or turned them down to reduce the feedback and ringing. Either the appliances are in and on and Peter complains that Laura is shouting all the time, or they are not working and Laura complains that she has to repeat everything. Toward the end of our time together I asked Peter if he would have any advice to offer someone who had just found out that they had PD. He ventured, "I'd say maybe you ought to go [to a neurologist], if you didn't have a doctor already. I've always had a lot of faith in my family doctor, but sometimes I think he thinks he knows it all and then he doesn't. But how do I know? It seems like they got a little pride, too. Don't you think?"

Laura added, "I've always been sorry that we didn't go to a neurologist when you first started those tremors. When those tremors first started in your right hand. I'm sorry we didn't go *then* to a neurologist to find out what that was." To Laura's mind, precious time had been wasted in waiting for their family doctor to agree that Peter had PD and to prescribe symptom-relieving treatment. Both Peter and Laura knew that something was wrong, but their trust in a family doctor dissuaded them from seeking another opinion. Peter lived with considerable untreated disability for almost five years. Because of it, he retired early and they moved. In many ways, Laura was right. Just a month or so after we met, care for Peter had become too difficult for Laura to manage alone, and Peter moved into a nursing home. He died within the year.

The Diagnostic Process

The disease/illness construct frames biology as the producer of a disorder and culture as the determinant of its outward, discernible expression (Kleinman 1988b). The diagnostic process ties these two realms of experience together, and embodiment can be viewed as the language through which the somatic and the larger cultural contexts of experience communicate. In the clinical encounter, diagnosis is a process of interpretation. It is the practice by which a medical practitioner translates the patient's subjective experience into medically recognized categories (Kleinman 1988a). PD's heterogeneity and its convergence with social and physiological signs of aging test the ease with which biomedical practitioners can readily identify the source of their patients' complaints.

Arriving at a PD diagnosis requires that sufferers identify their somatic complaints as something other than normal aging and that their health care providers agree with this assessment. The overlap of PD symptoms and signs of normal older age make this identification difficult, as is apparent from this list:

Constipation	Loss of sexual response
Anxiety	Slowness (cognitive and motor)
Depression	Stooped posture
Fatigue	Shuffling gait
Weakness	Tremor
Anhedonia	Memory lapses
Falling	Staid expression

The majority of the Iowa PD sufferers whom I met first seek the opinion of their general practitioner, who may see only a dozen or so cases of PD in their entire practice. Thus, in some ways patients are at the mercy of their family doctor's ability to identify PD (or their doctor's willingness to refer them to another specialist for further evaluation). The time between the first inkling that something is amiss and the receipt of a PD diagnosis can be lengthy, and the process often involves several health care providers—each with their own examinations, opinions, and fees. The answer Clifford, a seventy-year-old PD sufferer, gave when I asked him to describe PD is illustrative: "Well, I would say that you start out by shaking and it takes a little while to find out what it is for sure."

In general, an individual asks for a diagnosis to gain a sense of control, and in contemporary American discourse, a measure of personal closure. Patients also embark on this translation of the embodied into culturally recognizable forms of somatic disorder to legitimize themselves as sick and to access potential treatments (Iezzoni 2003). These positively valued outcomes are tempered by the stigma that certain disorders, such as AD or HIV, bestow on a patient. And, as discussed in chapter 1, the belief that suffering will end with the arrival of a diagnosis is commonly shattered when a life-altering disorder such as PD is pronounced.

At the outset of fieldwork, I was very much focused on how stereotypes about aging come to influence elders' interpretation of the body. The paths to diagnosis and its conveyance were located at the center of my inquiries. I would ask, "How did you know that something was wrong?" or "Were you satisfied with your doctor's opinion that it was just old age?" As I learned more about the complexity of diagnosing PD from a clinical perspective, I realized that in many cases it makes sense that providers wait until more severe or numerous symptoms emerge before divulging their suspicions. I also came to understand that PD sufferers' paths to diagnosis were almost as varied as the sufferers themselves.

Over time I recognized that the embodiment of aging had less to do with the diagnostic moment than it did with how people come to experience life after diagnosis, as aging PD sufferers.

Clinical Criteria for PD Diagnosis

PD is one condition in a set of disorders collectively known as parkinsonism. Some call idiopathic PD "Parkinson's syndrome" because they recognize that it may not be a single disease (Sethi 2003). It is also referred to as "L-Dopa responsive parkinsonism" (Meara 2000; Thomas and Dick 1998). PD can be distinguished from other parkinsonisms by the remittance of symptoms in the presence of dopaminergic medications. Rapidly developing imaging techniques such as positron emission tomography (PET) scans hold promise to improve diagnostic accuracy, but definitive diagnosis is only post mortem. PD diagnosis remains grounded in a clinical examination. Clinicians, advocacy organizations, and health care systems possess varying standards for differential diagnosis among parkinsonisms.

The classification criteria for PD are important for both practitioners and patients because they provide a prognosis and a treatment strategy (Foltynie, Brayne, and Barker 2002). Early diagnosis and treatment has been associated with longer disease-related life expectancy (Tanner and Ben-Shlomo 1999). Classification models for PD are variously based on a patient's age at onset, motor symptoms involved, rate of progression, type of cognitive involvement, underlying pathology, family history and genetics, occupational exposures, or history of head trauma (Foltynie, Brayne, and Barker 2002; Lewis et al. 2005; Meara and Bhowmick 2000). Age of onset can be used as a predictor of cognitive impairment and prognosis. The chronological cut-offs for the groups vary somewhat. Juvenile onset PD occurs before the second decade of life, young onset PD occurs between age twenty-one and the fourth or fifth decade, and late onset is variously defined as onset after age forty or seventy (Foltynie, Brayne, and Barker 2002; Meara and Bhowmick 2000). The usual onset of PD occurs during the sixth decade. Early onset PD tends to present slowly with predominant motor impairment, namely tremor. Later/normal onset PD progresses more quickly and has a greater impact on gait and postural reflexes (Meara and Bhowmick 2000). A small portion of all PD cases has been traced to genetic inheritance and a family history of PD.

In the biomedical world, the accuracy of PD diagnosis depends upon the stringency of inclusion criteria (Sethi 2003). Estimates of diagnostic accuracy range from 65 to 80 percent (Foltynie, Brayne, and Barker 2002; Lewis et al. 2005). When persons misdiagnosed with PD receive an accurate diagnosis, it is usually multiple system atrophy (MSA), progressive supranuclear palsy (PSP), AD, or vascular parkinsonism (Foltynie, Brayne, and Barker 2002). The United Kingdom Parkinson's Disease Society Brain Bank Clinical Diagnosis Criteria identifies PD on the basis of bradykinesia and one of the following symptoms—rigidity, resting tremor, or postural instability (Sethi 2003). Others argue that any two of the four symptoms are sufficient for positive diagnosis (Rodnitzsky 2000), and still others favor a more restrictive diagnosis that depends upon the presence of resting tremor, rigidity, and akinesia (Duvoisin and Sage 1996). Complicating these opinions on diagnostic criteria are the similarities among PD symptoms, normal age-related changes, symptoms of other age-related conditions, and larger societal beliefs regarding aging as a process of inevitable decline. The normal aging process causes postural changes and slows reflexes in ways similar to the results of PD (Rajput, Rajput, and Rajput 2003). Slowed motor function and rigidity may look like arthritis, and depression or cognitive slowness may be misdiagnosed as dementia. In the United States, often our understanding of senescence blinds us to recognizing PD (Brod, Mendelsohn, and Roberts 1998). We may erroneously equate slowed and stooped gait or hand tremor with "normal" aging or essential tremor.

The competing goals and values of research consortia, advocacy organizations, and pharmaceutical companies produce the various models for establishing a diagnosis of idiopathic PD. While this competition may be healthy from a scientific perspective, fostering an exchange of ideas and theories which may contribute to a better understanding of the underlying disease mechanism, from the sufferer's perspective it may serve to provide a false sense of hope. Indeed, sufferers who are loath to accept a PD diagnosis can pursue these competing frameworks to extend their search for a "better" diagnosis.

However practitioners may define it, the diagnosis of PD is a life-changing event, especially when one considers that the disease is progressive and degenerative. As discussed in chapter 1, Pinder (1990, 1992) demonstrates that the meaning of diagnosis differs for the PD affected and their physicians. For biomedical practitioners, whose professional goal is the diagnosis, arriving at a PD diagnosis may be prestige enhancing. It is a moment of coherence: The mystery is solved. Doctors in Pinder's study considered age of onset a factor in the gravity of the diagnosis; they judged PD a more somber diagnosis to give to middle-aged adults than to elders. In their view, elders had already lived most of their lives, so it was *lucky* that they were diagnosed in older age.

But for patients, diagnosis may be where the mystery begins. It is a space of incoherence. PD sufferers in Pinder's work characterized diagnosis as a life crisis that intensified feelings of being old, and a PD diagnosis made them feel "cheated by life" (Pinder 1992).

Old Age, Parkinson's, and the Diagnostic Process

A multitude of variables—age of onset, order and severity of symptoms, prior knowledge of PD, chance encounters with other PD patients, an article or television special, or a routine medical visit on an unrelated matter—converge to create a critical mass which produces engagement with the medical system. Once this critical mass exists and one entered the medical fray, for study participants, obtaining a PD diagnosis took anywhere from one visit to six years (see figure 2). During that time, they were variously diagnosed with and treated for essential tremor, arthritis, AD, and depression. And, of course, a small number of sufferers were told that they had "old age," nothing to worry about.

Diagnostic criteria impact patients in deeply personal ways. In many cases, study participants spent months wondering if they should seek a medical opinion on their symptoms, worrying that they would be wasting the doctor's time and that their symptoms were simply products of aging. At the prompting of friends and family, and by their internal "gut feeling" that something was amiss, elders sought their family doctor's advice. Regardless of age, the average length of time between onset of symptoms and receiving a PD diagnosis was a year and a half. The typical pattern was for sufferers to experience a subtle tremor in a finger or hand, seek their family doctor's advice, be referred to a neurologist, and then receive a diagnosis of PD from that specialist. Yet, only about half the participants experienced tremor first, and 15 percent of participants never developed a tremor. Instead, this group experienced balance problems, slowness, fatigue, depression, a sense of heaviness in their feet or head, a shuffling walk, or a lack of arm swing when walking.

The assessment of a pattern among diagnostic trajectories is complicated by the retrospective nature of narrative data. A single symptom may have been

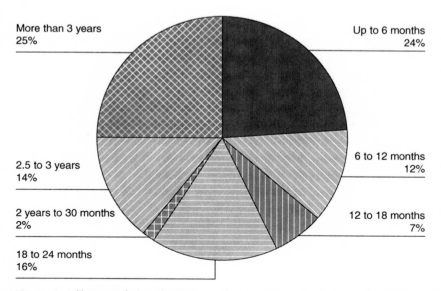

FIGURE 2 Self-reported time from onset of symptoms to diagnosis with Parkinson's disease

enough to drive a participant to seek medical advice, but looking back with the knowledge of a PD diagnosis, all of them could identify many symptoms of PD that at the time they had not identified as problematic. A tremor may have inclined a participant to seek care who at the time did not recognize their fatigue and stiffness as signs of something serious or as related symptoms of an underlying condition. Only after diagnosis were these symptoms read as PD related.

All PD sufferers come to their doctor with a unique set of symptoms of varying severity and order of appearance, at different ages, and with different rates of progression. PD's heterogeneity is clinically complex. Accordingly, all PD advocacy organizations in the United States stress the importance of seeing a neurologist who specializes in PD or movement disorders. For many Americans, access to these specialists is controlled by the gate-keeping function of their primary care physician. Many of the elder Iowans with whom I worked have lived in the same county for the entirety of their lives and have longstanding relationships with their physicians. When a referral isn't proffered, patients feel uncomfortable asking their family doctor for one, describing it as an implicit critique of their doctor's care. In the end, neurologists had diagnosed the vast majority of patients, and 90 percent of sufferers were receiving ongoing care from a neurologist. The remaining 10 percent were diagnosed by and received care from either an internist or a general practitioner. Interestingly, four persons were originally diagnosed by their chiropractor and subsequently sought a neurologist's opinion.

Being Seen

As I gathered sufferers' stories about how they came to know that they had PD, the differing perspectives on diagnosis held by physicians and sufferers became clear. PD diagnosis, in many ways, is about seeing. At onset, sufferers must first recognize that something out of the ordinary is occurring. Once they "see" that a particular symptom may warrant medical attention, they seek the advice of their family doctor, who must apprehend the patient's complaints as medical ones. The family doctor then interprets patients' complaints as old age, PD, or another disorder. Patients suspected of having PD are then most commonly referred to a neurologist for verification of the diagnosis or for further testing. Unfortunately, a commonality among many of the narratives was family physicians' failure to disclose their suspicions to their patients. Patients very often went to see the neurologist with a scant framework for interpreting the experience.

The neurological exam is a turning point at which sufferers learn to see their bodies in a new way. Neurologists obtain a medical history and gather vital signs, but they also ask patients to perform a number of activities that demonstrate mobility or balance impairment. Patients may be asked to touch their finger to their nose, to walk back and forth across a room, to resist their doctor's hands pushing them over, to draw a circle or write a sentence, or to hold their hands straight out in front of them. These examination techniques are employed to assess the presence of resting tremor, postural instability, lack of arm swing while walking, stride length, and micrographia—the small, cramped handwriting characteristic of PD. Neurologists also look at the patient's body for the stooped, forward-leaning posture associated with PD and at the patient's face to judge its relative expressivity. PD sufferers describe the exam as both alienating and thorough. To begin with, patients did not always understand why a neurologist was examining them or even what a neurologist was, and then they were asked to participate in a medical exam that to them felt like a series of tricks. More than one likened it to a roadside sobriety test, and one man called it a "dog and pony show." And after this bewildering experience, almost invariably, the neurologists summarily told the patients that they had PD, delivering the diagnosis with a brief commentary intended to be consoling but that PD sufferers frequently interpreted as insensitive.

Harold, a semiretired farmer in his early eighties, described these experiences in a conversation we had at his home. He had been living with tremor in one hand for a few years and had been told by two different physicians that it was nothing to worry about and perhaps related to an injury he had suffered in early adulthood. Harold never really believed that the injury and the shaking were related, but as the tremor was painless and did not get in the way of his farm duties, he didn't think much of it.

> At first I was [satisfied with the first diagnosis]. And then as time went by, I went to see [another physician] and he came up with the same diagnosis. And so two guys saying the same thing, why, you don't question it. A year went by, and I can't pinpoint what happened, but somewhere I am sure I read to go see a neurologist. So we went and made an appointment with [a neurologist at the hospital].
>
> I will tell you the only thing I remember that day; as usual we walked in and we sit down and we waited and waited and finally he came in. He said, "Get up and walk over to that door and turn around and come back." We hadn't discussed very much or anything. I thought, "Well, gosh. I am sure not having any trouble walking." So I gingerly started over to the door. I took two steps and he said, "Turn around and come back. You've got PD." His bedside manner was out of this world.

His wife asked Harold, "Didn't he also tell you to touch your nose?" And Harold replied, "Yes. And remember he waved his finger around?" She added, "And also he moved his arm around and different things." When I smiled knowingly during this exchange Harold asked me, "That doesn't surprise you?" I replied, "Well, he probably wanted to see that your eyes were coordinated, that you could follow things with your eyes. He would have wanted to feel your arm to see if it felt 'ratchety.'" Harold looked at me, exasperated: "Wouldn't that have been nice, if he had told me that? Doctors don't tell you anything. But anyway, he didn't say much more. But his bedside manner improved 100 percent, shortly thereafter. He said, 'Do you want the good news?' And I said, 'After what you just give me, I will take any good news you got.' "'Well, you waited until you were [in your seventies] to get it.'"

Harold's experience is not uncommon. With a reluctance perhaps not unique to Iowan elders, many felt that to question their physician's procedures was to offer an implicit critique. Thus they endured these unsatisfying and alienating encounters in quiet reflection and anticipation. Almost every narrative discussed the diagnostic process as a frustrating, sometimes mystifying experience. Edna, a PD sufferer in her early seventies, explains how her family doctor responded to her diagnosis. "They don't seem to know what causes it or anything. And when I went to [my doctor] I said, 'Well, what can I expect?' And he says, 'I'm no magician!' I thought that was a pretty poor answer." There is likely no pleasant way to convey to someone that they have PD, but the casualness with which doctors delivered the news surprised me, as it angered or depressed the persons to whom it had happened. PD sufferers are commonly taken aback by both the news and the way they are told.

Across narratives, doctors gave four main types of consolation with the diagnosis, each with its own well-intentioned and unintended offense. As in Harold's case, doctors might tell someone, "You have PD, but it's not so bad because you are already old." Even though Harold took this to be good news, the implication is that older people have less valuable lives, that their quality of life is less important, or that getting a disorder in later life is somehow less terrible than getting it in younger life. Reverse ageism appeared in one case, where a doctor asked a man in his fifties, "You are a little young to have PD, aren't you?" Another theme revolved around medicines, with several sufferers explaining that their doctor asked them if they could afford to spend so many dollars a month on a medicine. For example, on referring the patient to a neurologist for verification, one family doctor said, "I want to be sure, because it means that you are going to be on an expensive medication for the rest of your life." The final two themes of consolation in diagnosis centered on progression and prognosis. When Helen said to her doctor, "PD? People end up in the nursing home with PD." He replied, "Well, oh yeah, but that won't happen for a long time yet." And other sufferers reported that their doctors had assured them that their cases were "slow movers," that they shouldn't worry about the diagnosis because they had a mild case. How their neurologist was able to predict the course of a new case at diagnosis is unclear, but the hope that such words provided patients was not.

Receiving a PD diagnosis is often the end of a long process of wondering what might be going wrong and of patients looking for some explanation for their unusual symptoms. But, consistent with Pinder's (1990, 1992) study on PD and others' work on chronic illness in general (Charmaz 1983), participants' reactions to diagnosis rarely included relief, and frequently a greater sense of incoherence. As I recognized several months into fieldwork, diagnosis is not an endpoint but an initiating moment of interest for how PD influences the embodiment of aging in later life. A PD diagnosis is one of unknowing. There is a name for the disease, but no cure and little homogeneity. The treatments provide some symptomatic relief but leave much to be desired. It is the beginning of unknowing for many people. As they learn about PD and what it may or may not do to their ability to remain the selves they cherish and the selves they aim to be in retirement, their bodies are simultaneously becoming more alien and uncontrollable.

Virginia was in her midsixties when she for the first time understood that the way she saw herself was not consistent with the way others perceived her: "I was a little disappointed, I always say, [at] his bedside manner when he presented it to me. . . . He gave me the examination. [He was] a little blunt, which I thought was a little not good. And he said, 'You don't have a pinched nerve. You have PD.' He comes right out [and says]. I said, 'Well, what do you mean? Isn't there a blood test or a urine test or something?' 'No, it's just the trained eye of a neurologist.' It's true, which I didn't know [at the time]."

Virginia's interpretation of the diagnosis encounter reveals a moment when she understands that her estimation of her appearance and bodily control does not match the reality others perceive. For years Virginia's family had teased her for never smiling in photographs and for looking so serious all the time. In speaking with me, she reflected on how she made the connection between this subtle observation and the development of PD. At the time, she considered her family's comments unremarkable. After diagnosis, she realized that the flat demeanor they had teased her about was a sign of PD. Thus for some people, diagnosis brings with it a cascade of "Aha!" moments, times when the self as conceived is shown to be only distantly related to the self apprehended. Such a discord intensifies sufferers' feelings of loss and lack of control.

Life after Diagnosis

A significant part of diagnosis seeking involves seeing the body in a new way. First, elders must see their symptoms as abnormal, as I have noted, and then they must begin, to an extent, to see themselves as their physicians do: with stiff masked faces, stooped posture, and an indeterminate prognosis. One major aspect of developing this new vision of the self is establishing a relationship with a neurologist and seeking information about PD.

A majority of PD sufferers with whom I spoke continued to see the diagnosing neurologist for their long-term PD care. Despite their brusque and offputting communication styles, neurologists were seen as efficient, smart, busy, and professional. Participants held them in high esteem and derived a measure of self-worth from associating with persons of such high social status. PD patients proudly explained to me that their physician's "busyness" was a sign of quality. If it was hard to get an appointment, that means that he or she was in demand and thus a good doctor. Ultimately, in sufferers' eyes, good neurologists conducted PD research, took the time to explain things to their patients, and kept their patients apprised of new medications and potential side effects. They were thorough and methodical, did not prescribe too many medications, and sometimes helped people to obtain less expensive medicines from Canada.

Not everyone liked their original neurologist, and there were a dozen or so PD sufferers who had consulted several doctors. Some people did so because they did not believe that they had PD. Other sufferers complained that their neurologist did not seem to take patients' concerns *seriously*. According to PD sufferers, these neurologists did not listen to what their patients had to say, they rushed their patients through the exam, they did not return phone calls, or they prescribed medicines with intolerable side effects. The practice of seeking second opinions or finding a better neurologist was influenced by the local reputations of various neurology clinics and the alternately cold and clinical or charismatic and engaging neurologists who worked there. With a few exceptions, the PD support groups shared informal recommendations for PD care. Local neurologists, even if they were associated with internationally renowned neurologists in PD research, were sometimes viewed as inferior to the PD clinic a few hour's drive away. There are five neurology clinics with nationally recognized PD or movement disorder specialists within a five-hour drive from virtually anywhere in eastern Iowa. Patients who disagreed with their PD diagnosis or who felt that their treatment plan was inadequate sought the attentions of these popular practitioners.

Patients wanted more aggressive treatment, with newer medications, and they wanted a neurologist who acknowledged and treated all their symptoms. Interestingly, while avid information seekers grumbled about being their neurologists' "guinea pigs," they did so with some pride. Patients disliked having to constantly change their medication dosage and type, but they enjoyed being attended to carefully and were proud of their participation in clinical trials. Vernon's case provides a clear example of this. We were talking about the diagnostic process and how he came to understand that he was not just getting old. I had asked Vernon, then eighty-two, if he had been diagnosed by his family doctor and whether his general practitioner had referred him to a neurologist.

VERNON: I guess I was referred [to a neurologist]. I'm really on my third one now.

SAMANTHA: Your third neurologist?

VERNON: Yes. I guess I thought once I learned what it was I was surprised it wasn't worse, my symptoms weren't worse. I won't say that I'm disappointed because I'm missing something. [laughs]

The other two I, uh, I'm not too sure why—I never in my life changed doctors before—and that I'm kind of surprised as I look back on it. I just wasn't very pleased with what I was getting fed back. And I just got the feeling that, uh, neither of the original two people felt I was *serious* about this whole thing. I don't want to take potshots at somebody who is not here to defend themselves, and I wouldn't even name them or anything. But I felt that, well, this doctor that I'm with now is so superior in my judgment. I'm not a medic, so maybe I'm judging improperly. . . . But I felt that this was fairly serious and I wanted the best possible [care]—I guess everybody's selfish that way.

Vernon's neurologist was a popular one and considered superior because of his sense of humor, tendency to prescribe lower doses, and active program of research. I frequently overheard this neurologist's patients urging other sufferers to consult him for their care. In the eyes of some PD sufferers, to settle for one's hometown general practitioner was to resign oneself to suboptimal care, to the point some sufferers considered others as not taking care of themselves because they did not see a well-regarded specialist for their care.

From Diagnosis to Support

The second principle way sufferers develop a new vision of themselves is to gather information about PD, and one place this happened was in PD support groups. A common part of the consolation aspect of diagnosis was the doctor's providing new patients with the contact information for the local PD support group. Support groups function as resources for both caregivers and PD sufferers. Groups can help decrease social isolation and normalize the experience of PD. They provide information on PD research, on new therapies, or on other age-related services and issues; offer advice on how to cope with symptoms; and share tricks for relearning how to perform fine motor skills. I worked with thirteen different support groups, each with its own personality. Some groups focused on providing formal educational programs, whereas other groups emphasized the importance of informal resources and experience sharing among attendees. Opinions as to the value of support groups can be characterized by three attitudes: support groups normalize the experience of PD, support groups make you appreciate the abilities that you still have, and support groups show you what you have to "look forward to."

Notably, more than half the support groups were started by PD sufferers who wanted a community. They needed to learn more about PD and wanted to know that they were not alone. These groups are spaces where PD's otherwise stigmatizing presentation is acceptable and, to an extent, normalized, as is apparent in these comments from Anthony, who is sixty-five:

> I think that one of the biggest things that helps me is the support group.
> Because things that I've been keeping inside me about what happens to

me, that nobody knows, I'm hearing somebody else say they have the same problem. And you don't feel like a weirdo. You probably know quite a bit about PD. You can be talking, your speech just stops. People look at you. Thinking that I'm going to pick that pen up, by the time I get there I could forget what I wanted. It's strange, and it's really more strange when you're—see there, I lost my train of thought. I lost it right there. So, it's a good example.

For Anthony, the support group was a place to "let it all hang out." And when I sat at a table flanked by people in wheelchairs, with walkers, with shaking hands and nodding heads, it was easy to recognize the camaraderie inherent in such a social space.

People in the second category, who felt that support groups helped them to "keep things in perspective," shared this positive view of support groups. I was talking with David, seventy-seven, a retired mechanic, about why he went to a support group.

SAMANTHA: What do you feel are the benefits of going to the meeting?

DAVID: The benefit? Just the idea that if you think you've got it bad, there are people there who've got it a lot worse than you. At least we know someone else has it. That's important to us.

SAMANTHA: Would you say that you are an optimist or a pessimist?

DAVID: Oh, I am an optimist. You know, you feel sorry for them people. You think you got it bad, well they've *really* got it bad. Makes you feel a little better.

Several people mentioned that, compared to other patients, they didn't have it "too bad." Those who have "really got it bad" were PD sufferers who had severe dyskinesia or obvious cognitive impairments. In the hierarchy of disability, losing control over your body is relative, and losing control of your mind was the worse fate. The feeling was that not only did the cognitively impaired have PD, but also they no longer knew how poorly they were doing: They didn't realize that they were the objects of pity.

Not everyone I met attended a support group. Those who did not were the most likely to hold the third opinion, that people who attended support groups were too fixated on their disease or were extremely disabled and depressing to be around. As one eighty-year-old PD sufferer explained: "I've had PD a long time. I hope it continues to progress slowly. I don't enjoy attending the support group. Seeing others that are worse off is a letdown. All of this so-called research they tell about never seems to reach me." Such people see support groups as depressing and a waste of time. Some PD sufferers avoided the support group because they didn't want to be around people with dementia or impairments worse than their own. Bonnie, sixty-three, told me before she found a support group with better programming: "For a while I didn't want anybody to know. For a little bit, I tried to hide it. And then I thought, 'This is crazy. What difference does it make if they know that I have this?' So then we let people know. . . . We went to one support group meeting, where all of the cases there were very severe and the program didn't offer any help in any way. It was a very depressing situation. I thought, 'We aren't going to do this anymore.'"

Those who were avid support group attendees argued that support groups needed the people who didn't need *them*. In other words, support groups desired members who could demonstrate that PD served as a condition that can influence life, not a life sentence.

The findings of Charlton and Barrow (2002) reinforce this last theme. The coping strategies of PD support group members were compared to those of nonattendees. Attendees used their group participation as a point of social comparison; they were able to view their own circumstances as relatively less burdensome compared to those of other group members with more severe PD-related limitations. Support group members discussed the importance of learning to live one day at a time, maintain a positive attitude, work toward self-acceptance, and approach with a "fighting spirit" conditions PD placed upon them. In contrast, those sufferers who did not attend a group "acknowledged PD, but did not seek to adapt their lives to accommodate it any more than was absolutely necessary" (477).

Being Diagnosed with a Condition

Being diagnosed with a condition locates a beginning rather than an endpoint. It may be a momentary pause in the search for a cause for suffering, but the lack of consensus regarding diagnostic criteria and prognosis underscores the shift from biographical disruption to lifelong condition. Sufferers are generally dismayed by the diagnosis and experience a period of coming to terms with what having PD might mean for their identity, family, and future. Yet, this biographical disruption fades in importance as sufferers come to experience PD as neither disease nor normal aging.

PD disrupts the essential values of the archetypal American self— independence, autonomy, individualism, self-control, and self-efficacy. Its progressive, deteriorating impact on the body threatens sufferers' self-concept. Sufferers' inability to engage in the activities that make them human in their particular communities leads others to view them with suspicion. This suspicion coincides with a time in life when a certain degree of limitation is considered acceptable and normal. Such a coincidence of social processes presents elder PD sufferers with two differing modes of embodying somatic phenomena. They interpret and make sense of the body through the competing and overlapping idioms of aging and disease progression, and ultimately come to experience

PD as a condition which accelerates, mediates, and obscures aging, as the following chapters explore.

The diagnostic trajectory for PD is predicated upon the task of separating signs of normal aging from those of the disease. Because early symptoms of PD overlap with those commonly assigned to aging, arriving at a PD diagnosis can be a lengthy process. While not all PD sufferers read their symptoms as normal signs of aging, and others knew from onset that they had probable PD, after diagnosis sufferers' embodiment of the disorder is shaped by their beliefs about aging. Inasmuch as diagnosis is about seeing, naming, and authorizing certain behaviors, it is also a reflection of what it means to grow older. From diagnosis on, the questioning of embodiment is transformed and somatic experience is identified as PD-related or not. Whatever led up to diagnosis, after it had been conferred no one attributed PD to normal old age. But receiving a PD diagnosis profoundly alters sufferers' sense of being old. As individual sufferers come to make sense of what the disorder means for them, they realize that differentiating aging from PD is not easy. When asked to define the difference, they find that the boundaries evade identification. As Clifford, whose words title this chapter, patiently told me: "Well, I would say that you start out by shaking and it takes a little while to find out what it is for sure." Like aging, PD is a condition whose meaning is elucidated over time—the time from the earliest inklings of somatic disorder to diagnosis, the time from one plateau of impairment to the next, the incapacitating times between medication doses and the wondering how much longer they will work, and the time of unknowing ahead.

4

It's a Nasty, Hiding Disease

Introduction: No One's Going to Buy Into This Situation

It was more than fifteen years ago when Helen noticed her legs shaking whenever she was seated. She casually mentioned it to her family doctor, who suggested that she see a neurologist. At first the neurologist diagnosed it as essential tremor and sent her on her way with no information on prognosis, no relief for symptoms, and no plan for follow up. When Helen's symptoms became so severe that she spent hours sitting with her legs curled up and rocking back and forth to relieve the uneasy feeling in her legs, she returned to the neurologist for more information and some relief. At that point, his assessment of her disorder changed and he informed her that she had PD. Helen was incredulous, as we saw in chapter 3, asking him, "PD? People end up in the nursing home with PD." His impersonal reply—"Well, oh yeah, but that won't happen for a long time yet"—contributed to her sense of despair about the future and her shock at having coming down with a condition that she considered something "for old people." She was fifty years old.

Despite her reservations about her doctor's bedside manner, Helen continued to see this neurologist for almost five years, during which time she tried numerous PD medications. Her frustration with ineffective medications and her unresponsive physician reached a tipping point when he refused to acknowledge that her unremitting fatigue might be part of the disease process. Her doctor was focused on reducing tremor; Helen was intent on reducing her fatigue. Her physician's inability to align his concerns with her own led her to seek out a new neurologist, who both validated her experience of PD and established an effective medication regimen for her—one that includes a prescription not legally available in the United States.

Ten years ago she and her husband moved into a ranch-style condominium to relieve themselves of the responsibilities of their large house. Helen still misses her lavish perennial gardens, but diminished stamina and strength made it hard for her to maintain the beds to her satisfaction. She explains, "I could work from dawn to dusk in the yard. I was having more trouble doing that and I was falling down a lot. I didn't have the energy I needed to take care of [my garden]. . . . It's increasingly difficult to do that kind of thing because I am so stiff. And also because if I lean too far forward I fall on my face. Too far back and I am sitting on the ground. Or else I get down and I can't get up. Fortunately, my neighbors all know what's wrong with me or they'd think I'd taken to drink!" She laughs.

Helen's outward demeanor, though stiff at times, is one of ebullience and cheer. She has an intensive support network of neighbors who check in to see if she needs help with anything—and who do so more frequently since the death of her husband several years ago. Helen is a self-described "career woman" and it is important to her to feel occupied and productive. She is an avid reader and letter writer, and maintains friendships with a number of people across the country. She still grieves for her beloved husband but has adjusted to living alone and enjoys the freedom of being able to come and go as she pleases. "I actually have days, more and more, where I say, 'Who said [that I have to clean the house today]?' I don't want to do this, this, and this first. I want to read this book.' I will spend hours in here just sitting and reading a book. And I think to myself, 'Aren't you lucky?' "

Over the past decade Helen's medication dosages have steadily crept upward as her function has steadily decreased. When we met, she was taking medicine every three hours and suffering from restless legs, intermittent dyskinesia, fatigue, tremor, and slowness. I asked her, "What is PD for you?"

> I am shaking now. That will be whether its pleasurable excitement or stress, which makes it happen. Probably the tremor, now, as far as comfort is concerned, is the most uncomfortable part. If I were up moving around, the tremor wouldn't be that obvious, you know. Not to mention I don't know what time it is [checks time]. I could probably nibble on a pill by now.
>
> It's the frustration of not being able to do what I've always been able to do. I said to you earlier, it's not safe for me to get on the stepstool. If I want to dust the drapery above the kitchen sink, well, I have to climb the stepstool and have one foot on the stepstool and one foot in the sink in order to reach it—which never used to be a problem. Now I wouldn't dare to do that. I went to get the mail, when we had all that snow, and I tried to straddle the snow. I've learned that I don't want to get straddle-legged, because now I can't move at all! The back foot won't move; the front foot won't move. There you are straddling the snowdrift, thinking, "Oh, good. I'm going to be sitting down in the street in the snow in a minute."

The rigidity and the tremor give me a lot of trouble. I don't know how much help the medication is as far as the rigidity and the balance are concerned. I know that I am more rigid. At one point my energy was so low that I would just lay down where I was. I'd be in the midst of shopping and realize that I wasn't functioning, that I was just doddering around, thinking, "Can you get back home?" I'd come home, go back to sleep for an hour, go back and finish what I was doing. . . .

It feels like it's a jolt of electricity sometimes. I've had a lot of trouble with that lately. 'Long about eight o'clock at night, I'll have done fine all day long, and I'll just be sitting and reading and all of the sudden it will just be like, zzzzz. "Oh, no. Not you again." And then the leg will start going. I think, "What is that?" You know, if you could see it on camera, it would probably be amusing. It doesn't feel amusing. It's like the St. Vitus dance! There would be no way, if I were in public, that I could hide it. . . . That is probably the worst symptom I have. I am sure it must come from the PD. I don't know what else it might be. It is totally consuming.

We spoke at length about the medications she has tried, the neurologists she's consulted, and the ongoing relinquishment of control over her body. She continued:

It's a pain in the butt. Is it an illness or is it a disability? I guess its both. I have been very independent and liked it that way. It has robbed me of that independence. If I could actually physically locate the thing [PD], I would probably punch it [laughs]. Because I have to ask for help so much, and I really, really resent that. . . . Sometimes it will be like every day there is something more restricted. . . . Well, people talk about their feet freezing to the floor; I haven't had that happen but a few times. What I have is my brain locking. I call it brain lock. It really does. I am doing something, mentally, and I run into a problem or don't understand something right away; then anxiety sets in and I freeze and I can't do it. I just get more and more frustrated and confused. I have learned to leave it alone and come back to it.

[Parkinson's has] stolen my sense of security and my independence. I don't know if I would have those thoughts otherwise, at least not this soon. People say that when you lose those around you, you begin thinking of your own mortality. . . . But only from the later years of the PD have I thought about it on a personal level. . . . I like to be where things are comfortable and pretty. I am not ready to give up my stuff! I like all my stuff and it's not going to fit into a nursing home. I have enough trouble getting to the bathroom on time without having to turn on a light and the nurse not getting there to help me, or soiling myself. I don't want to do that. Nobody wants to do that. You basically go through life not thinking about that happening to you. Really, the concept of dying is just so impossible to grasp. You can't comprehend what that means. And people with religion are comforted by that and I am grateful that they are. But it doesn't do that for me. It doesn't seem too logical. . . . Not long ago somebody said to me, "You should be out and about. You are still young and attractive. You could still have a love life." I thought, "Have you lost your mind? Nobody is going to buy into this situation!"

A clear demonstration of how PD functions as a condition on aging is Helen's comment, "I don't know if that I would have those thoughts otherwise"; for Helen, an intelligent women in her sixties, having PD meant being restricted, not having intimate relationships, and an inevitable decline. PD has accelerated her aging because it has made her confront death, long-term care, and having to ask for help at a younger age than she anticipated. She identifies such circumstances as part of growing older, but she is not yet ready to be old.

What Is Parkinson's Disease? Biomedical and Sufferer Explanations

Biomedical Explanations

Parkinson's was first described in 1817 by the physician James Parkinson, who called it the "shaking palsy." As described in chapter 1, it is a chronic, progressive disease of the central nervous system that primarily affects motor function, but that in the later stages can progressively affect the autonomic nervous system (Jankovic 2003). The pathophysiology of PD is complex. The symptoms of PD are thought to be the result of the death of dopaminergic neurons in the area of the brain that coordinates motor function, the substantia nigra (Kirschstein 2000; Youdim and Riederer 1997). These neurons of the substantia nigra provide dopamine to the forebrain, which regulates emotion, and to the middle brain (the corpus striatum), which is involved with motor function. When approximately 80 percent of the dopamine-producing neurons have been destroyed, the balance between the two neurotransmitters which control motor function, dopamine and acetylcholine, becomes skewed and motor symptoms emerge (Curtis and McDonald 1998). The pathophysiology of PD overlaps with other age-related conditions such as Lewy body disease, Pick's disease, and AD, and with normal age-related changes in brain anatomy. The ultimate source of this pathology in most PD cases is unknown; a majority of PD sufferers have idiopathic cases.

Basic science research into the mechanisms that cause neuronal death in PD is complemented by a broad literature that examines PD as a public health issue with substantive quality of life decline. People with chronic conditions are more likely to have psychological distress (Verhaak et al. 2005), and such distress is associated with greater disability and a lower quality of life (Schrag 2004). To some extent, these conditions are endogenous to PD. Nonmotor symptoms of PD can include dementia, depression, anxiety, autonomic dysfunction or sleep disorders (Dewey 2003). Anhedonia, an inability to experience pleasure; abulia, the lack of ability to express free will or to make decisions; and anomia, an inability to identify the relationship between a word and an object, also co-occur with PD. Considering the limitations that PD can impose on the body and their related constraints on social or interpersonal engagement, the high coincidence of depression and anxiety with PD is unsurprising. In light of the age cohort of PD sufferers, it is also unsurprising that a substantial number of them eventually develop mild cognitive impairment or other dementia.

Sufferer Explanations

In addition to tremor, slowness, and rigidity, the people that I worked with in Iowa reported having numerous symptoms, including micrographia, constipation, anxiety, and slurred speech (see figure 3 for a summary of their reported symptoms). There was no relationship between PD symptoms and such variables as mode of embodiment, decade of life, MOS scale scores, or age at onset. There were few sex differences in symptom prevalence, either (see Solimeo 2008 for an in-depth discussion of sex and gender in regard to PD symptomatology). And, consistent with the literature, PD sufferers in this study fared worse than other

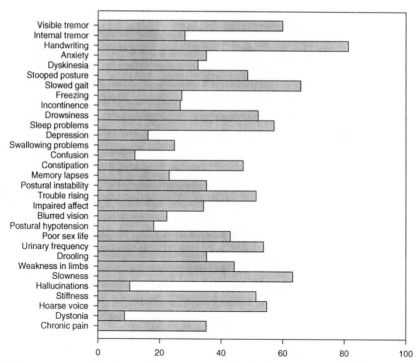

FIGURE 3 Percentage of questionnaire respondents reporting selected PD symptoms

older adults in the general population on every scale of the RAND MOS health measure. But sufferers' quality of life is linked not only to the presence of later life infirmities but to the larger social sphere in which they are experienced. Sufferer and caregiver descriptions of PD clearly illustrate this relationship.

Sufferers' definitions of PD are as varied as clinical ones. Almost half my interviewees could not define PD, saying, "I don't know," or "It's just a disease." About 20 percent provided a medical definition, such as "PD is a neurological disease affecting the dopamine in the brain." Roughly equal numbers of people defined PD as either a nerve, brain, or genetic disease. Finally, a few of the persons I interviewed explained that PD was a disease of the muscles or part of aging.

Being asked for a definition of PD seemed to make people ill at ease. They shifted in their chairs, qualified their responses with statements such as," I don't know if this is right," or "I've never had to explain it before." Their discomfort came from a fear of getting something wrong, but it also marked something significant about their experience: They didn't know what PD was or what to expect. In the end, most people defined PD in terms of the primary symptoms that functioned as conditions on their life experiences. PD was not so much a disease as a constraint derived from particular somatic limitations, and these limitations formed a context for their aging process.

A Condition Affecting Self-Control: Living with Shaking Hands

A popular PD joke, "How do you shake hands with a Parky? You just grab hold and hang on," indicates the ubiquity of the annoying and sometimes painful shaking associated with the disorder. Resting tremor is the predominant symptom in a majority of PD cases (Sethi 2003). Generally, tremor first appears on one side of the body and over time slowly progresses to engage the whole body. Tremor appears when the affected body part is at rest, and anxiety exacerbates its intensity. As Helen's comments indicate, both good stressors such as winning a game and negative stressors such as trying to make a left turn against traffic intensify tremor. Some people have a barely perceptible (to others) shaking, while others have no tremor at all. About half the study participants experienced tremor "often," and the majority (85 percent) had tremor at least occasionally. Tremor functions as a mark of membership and authentication, a shared condition affecting disparate lives. I overheard on several occasions remarks such as, "You have PD? Oh, you don't have a tremor." In a few cases, without the tremor to signal disease status, I could not guess which spouse had PD (in two instances it turned out that both husband and wife did).

When tremor was present, I found that I could use it as a rough gauge by which to measure how long someone had had PD. Newly diagnosed patients were more likely to try to disguise a tremor. They sat on their hands, held their shaking hand steady with their unaffected hand, and hid their shaking hand in their pocket or under their arm. Those who had been living with tremor for years seemed at times to no longer even notice it, sometimes to the detriment of our interview recordings, which were occasionally obscured by a rhythmic tapping on the microphone.

Tremor can become an all-consuming annoyance and source of pain, stress, and embarrassment. For tremor-dominant PD sufferers, shaking is synonymous with the disorder. Tremor is exhausting. Physically, it causes aches, soreness, and fatigue. It gets in the way of performing once-simple tasks such as buttoning a shirt, picking up a pill, or holding the newspaper steady enough to read. Shaking is an outward expression of sufferers' lack of control over their own bodies. It makes them suspect, their shaking limbs a sign to others that something is amiss.

PD sufferers' efforts to manage their shaking exhausts them in a social and interpersonal sense, too. Nijhof (1995) found that PD sufferers withdrew from social spheres because of tremor-related embarrassment. Participants in his study emphasized the separation of public and private spaces (or "dangerous" and "safe" spaces for deviance), and withdrew from social interactions that marked them as "deviant." Participants in my research echoed Nijhof's findings. People tried not to share hymnals or to shake hands in church, but in doing so risked drawing attention to their apparently unfriendly behavior. One woman admitted that she never used change to pay for things at a store: Getting the coins out of her purse was too embarrassing. Sufferers try to maintain their privacy and dignity by hiding or controlling the shaking hand and by continuing to partici-pate in their usual activities. This maintenance consumes extraordinary amounts of energy and is never seamless or complete. For instance, when I met Vernon, he had had PD for less than a year. He often hid his shaking hand when he was in public, perhaps not realizing that other people could still perceive the shaking as it traveled up his arm. In fact, this technique is short-lived: A handful of male PD patients admitted to me that other people had mistaken them for sex-ual deviants, interpreting their attempt to hide a shaking hand as masturbation.

A Condition Affecting Movement: Shuffling, Falling, and Freezing

Like tremor, gait problems signify loss of control over the body. The stooped posture and shuffling walk that accompany PD make people appear older and frailer than they feel, and the changes in gait coordination and speed serve as constant reminders that sufferers' independence is slowly slipping away. Walking and mobility are signifiers of independence in the United States, and mobility impairments profoundly impact sufferers' sense of bodily integrity and self-reliance. This may be particularly so among members of the rural commu-nities with whom I worked. Rural living often requires physical strength and stamina and mobility impairments threaten one's ability to contribute. Walking problems portend the possibility of relocation and the relinquishment of the family home and the roles and status that accompany it. Yet PD is not solely to blame for ambulatory impairments in later life. Age-related changes in weight, bone density, postural reflexes, and arthritis can cause elders' walk to become slower and stiffer and may cause their posture to become more rounded and inclined forward. Walking impairment is affected by pain from biomechanical causes, neurological problems, limited endurance, or missing limbs (Iezzoni 2003). PD worsens these problems with ambulation.

Parkinson's disease negatively affects ambulation in many ways. A stooped posture, shuffling walk, and loss of postural reflexes contribute to postural instability. Sufferers feel unsteady on their feet, take small mincing steps, and are more likely to fall (Jankovic 2003). They may appear drunk because of their uncoordinated and slowed gait. They may "freeze" in doorways, at cracks in the sidewalk, or at other disruptions in the walking surface. Everett, an eighty-one-year-old retiree, experienced freezing on a daily basis. He would approach a doorway and get stuck at the threshold, unable to get his feet to comply with his intention to pass through. In this situation, Everett reverted to his military training; he counted off steps and raised his knees high, as if marching in formation. He learned that this break in routine walking would interrupt the freeze and restore his motor function.

The shuffling steps so characteristic of PD cause many people to catch a toe on the smallest of bumps on the walking surface, resulting in falls. Unfortunately, many people with PD have a limited reflex to catch themselves; I saw a few terribly banged-up elders sporting facial lacerations, black eyes, and skinned arms. In a dark sort of irony, other PD patients are prone to festation, unable to keep their gait from accelerating when they wish, as referenced in this PD joke: "Good news! Next year the first annual Parkinson's Special Olympics will be held in Shaker Heights. The first year there will be four events: Free Falling, Vest Buttoning, Doorway Obstacle Course, and the Hundred-yard Shuffle (a second prize will be awarded in this event to the contestant who can stop first)." I did not understand the ramifications of festation until I saw Hazel wearing a large patch over one side of her face at a support group meeting. She had been walking along the sidewalk and her legs began to run way from her. It was all she could do to put up her arms to stop herself as she walked into a brick wall.

The negative impact of PD on the biomechanical aspects of walking is a source of shame and embarrassment. Several men shared stories with me that exposed their outrage at these changes. They no longer recognized their reflection in storefront windows; they wondered who these little old men with hunched backs were. Older men expressed resentment toward their mincing steps and missed the long, powerful strides of a youthful walk (Solimeo 2008). Their shortened strides, shuffling steps, curved backs, and omnipresent awareness of their vulnerability to falls and fractures intensifies their sense of being frail and ineffectual.

Sufferers such as June, eighty-four and divorced, took pains to avoid risky activities, but such precautions limited their sense of self-efficacy and optimism about the future. When I asked June to describe PD for me, her response focused on falling and risk management.

JUNE: Well, it is a progressive disease that affects your balance and your handwriting, which I miss. Your walking, definitely. You shuffle your feet instead of picking them up. You have to be very careful about falling. I haven't fallen now for, I'd say, over a year. I took three or four good falls and I am very, very careful. In living alone you have to be careful. Other things, too. For instance, I never turn the faucet on and leave the room.

SAMANTHA: Why is that?

JUNE: If I should fall before I came back, what would happen to the water? I would flood my apartment! [laughs].

June laughs at the possibility of falling while the tap is running, but there is an underlying sadness to her story as well. Her comments illustrate how the possibility and unpredictability of falling can influence the minutiae of everyday life.

Whether June's is a realistic fear may be debated; however, gait impairment is associated with considerable risk of falling, sustaining injuries, and nursing home placement. Falls and unintentional injuries are frequent incidents in PD sufferers' lives. Motor impairment, polypharmacy, and postural instability substantively increase PD patients' likelihood of falling. PD sufferers not only possess a propensity toward falling, but also motor impairment affects their ability to reflexively put out their arms to break a fall, and because of their age, PD sufferers have a greater probability of having coincident metabolic bone disorders (Fink et al. 2005), which dramatically increases their risk of fracture.

Clinical research on the incidence of falling and its sequelae among PD patients is informative. In a retrospective survey study of PD patients at a Midwestern PD clinic, more than half reported a fall in the past two years and about one-fifth of fallers sustained a fracture as a result of their fall (Wielinski et al. 2005). The authors determined that increased age, disease duration, dementia, and a diagnosis of atypical PD increased the risk of falling. A study of 109 PD patients conducted in the United Kingdom found an incidence of falls of 68 percent (Wood et al. 2002). I asked the PD sufferers with whom I worked to report whether they had fallen in the preceding month. Of questionnaire respondents, 37.8 percent had experienced a fall, and more than half (54.4 percent) reported that they incurred an injury from the fall. While those who reported an injury most often incurred only bumps and bruises (83 percent), about 10 percent suffered a fracture and the remainder required stitches.

The risk of injury from a fall is considerable, and it makes sense that PD sufferers take steps to avoid situations where a fall might be likely. Among all older adults, unintentional injury due to falls is an important source of mortality and morbidity (Fuller 1997; Lilley, Arie, and Chilvers 1995; Schoenfelder and Why 1997; Tinetti 1994). Falls accounted for 25.2 percent of nonfatal injuries treated in emergency departments in the United States in the year 2000 (National Center for Injury Prevention and Control 2001). Fractures, which are slower to heal in elders than in the general population, often require hospitalization, physical therapy, and prescription drugs, and produce restricted ambulation or mobility. And PD sufferers, because of their mobility limitations, may possess an even more reduced capacity for postfracture rehabilitation. More sobering are the emerging data on PD sufferers' potentially greater risk of also having osteoporosis, a metabolic bone disorder with its own associated risks for fracture and disability (Sato et al. 2001; Sato, Kikuyama, and Oizumi 1997; Wood and Walker 2005). While many PD patients are at risk of osteoporosis simply because of their age, several other mechanisms for increased risk are under study. These include deficiencies in vitamins D, K, or calcium, and the low bone mineral density associated with a lack of weight-bearing exercise (Fink et al. 2005).

A Condition Affecting the Speed of Life: Slowness

Even though bradykinesia, or slowness, is a diagnostic indicator of PD, it is likely the one most commonly interpreted as a symptom of old age. This slowness of movement affects both gross- and fine-motor skills. It contributes to a loss of automatic movements such as swallowing, blinking, maintaining balance, and expressing emotion or mood through facial affect. The reduction in these reflexes causes drooling, tearing, an increased likelihood of falls, a tendency toward choking, and the stiff expressionless gaze of PD sufferers. Bradykinesia can also cause aches and pains, cramps, burning or tingling feeling in the hands and feet, and stooped posture. Less socially acceptable to discuss is its effect on the gastrointestinal tract: Chronic constipation is one of the few universals among PD patients.

When slowness appeared as the initial symptom of PD, regardless of age participants did not recognize it as a medical issue. Several women thought that their slowness was attributable to arthritis or that their aches were symptoms of fibromyalgia. Spouses shared with me their guilt at having berated their partners for being lazy and apathetic—not realizing at the time that it was PD. Those who did seek a medical opinion on their slowness did so reluctantly, as the following comments from two eighty-year-old PD sufferers indicate.

SAMANTHA: When did you first start feeling like something was wrong?

HAZEL: Actually, I didn't. . . . The kids began to get concerned. They knew that I was more or less slow in whatever I did, but they said I was abnormally slow. [My husband finally] said, "Go to the doctor." And I said, "What do I tell him? That I'm slow?" Well, I went and I was slow. [laughs] Took her about ten minutes.

Well, outside of swallowing, and the slowness of gait, you know, I think I wouldn't have a problem with PD if I wasn't so tired all of the time. But that's also a symptom. And I don't mean just tired. I mean extremely tired, where it's an effort for you to do anything. . . . No, it isn't drowsy. It's the body. Because when I stand, it feels like there was nothing except water in my legs. You know, that I could very easily faint? But, the strange part of the whole thing is that I can get up in the morning. And the mornings that I feel tired and exhausted, and can hardly go, about two o'clock in the afternoon, or three, it'll all go away. And I'll feel real peppy. And it shouldn't be that way! [laughs] It should be that way after you after you get up in the morning. But I have no idea. I said to the doctor, I said, "I'm so extremely tired all the time." I said, "Is that a part, or a symptom?" He said yes. And [laughs] this is all the reply I get. But I wish there was something, a vitamin or something that you could take that would pep you up a bit.

Slowness may seem a benign sort of symptom, and even PD sufferers themselves would place its significance lower than that of, say, tremor or memory loss. But slowness can be a source of dissatisfaction and frustration. Sufferers who have akinetic, or tremorless PD, tend to experience the most severe bradykinesia. For them, slowness is not simply being unable to do things as quickly as they once did, it is the sapping of their energy, ambition, and self-efficacy. This kind of slowness is life changing. Slowness interferes with sufferers' ability to automatically perform the movements necessary to do simple things, such as pick up a pencil or move a hair away from in front of one's eyes.

People often remarked to me that their mind was perfectly fine, but their body was no longer listening. They would be sitting at the kitchen table reading a consent form and want to turn the next page. The process of separating the pages, lifting the top page over to the back, finding the corner of the packet, and smoothing over the seam formed by the staple could be agonizingly slow. After several instances in which interviewees struggled to manage the physical components of reading such forms, I elected to mail them a week ahead of our interview, to save them the indignity of nakedly demonstrating their slowed movements. At first glance slowness seems minor, but when you consider the additive effect of the impairment on the rhythm of daily life—rising from bed, dressing oneself, grooming, preparing and eating breakfast—basic activities take on a whole new weight and proportion of sufferers' energies. As a condition affecting will, slowness can both deter and preclude sufferers' ability to act on their desires.

One special aspect of slowness, decreased affect, presents a unique challenge. Decreased affect does not mean that PD sufferers are unable to smile or show expression, but that those affected must work to exaggerate what they think is an expression in order for other people to see it. This symptom is often recognized by family members and friends long before the afflicted can see the change in themselves. Virginia, who is sixty-six and was diagnosed with PD in her late fifties, remarked to me that her family began to complain that she never smiled in photographs, as we have seen. "Yes, that's one thing I noticed," she said. "In pictures I thought I was smiling nice and broad, but I was only [smiling] a little bit." Many people who notice the PD mask misinterpret it as expressing anger, disinterest, or depression. Harry, a congenial PD sufferer in his seventies, felt that his demeanor contributed to his and his wife's decreasing social circle. Historically, they have been active members of their community, participating in church activities, hosting neighborhood parties, and contributing countless hours to political activism at local, state, and national levels. But as Harry's PD progressed, other used the outward markers of his disease state—gait impairment and the mask—to exclude him from social events in which he has always participated. As he and his wife explained to me:

JENNIE: We do know where people decide that we can't do things. We aren't as much fun, though. You know? Right in the beginning one friend did say that he talked about it too much.

HARRY: And that wasn't even true.

JENNIE: Nobody wants to hear about it. You might have it, but don't talk about it. . . . I don't think people like to look at him.

HARRY: Maybe they think I am mad. It could be the mask.

JENNIE: Also, they . . . nobody wants to have something like that happen to them. I think watching when you can't walk or so forth. It makes them more nervous than it makes you.

HARRY: Yeah. I suppose. . . . I think the mask does intimidate people. They think I am mad. Angry.

My own experience with the mask is telling. As I described in chapter I, even though I knew that PD could decrease facial expression, I was initially intimidated by the mask. Facing stern expressions during interviews, I often had to remind myself to not take them personally. As anthropologists before me have discovered, learning the spoken language of your field site is only a small portion of communication. The nonverbal aspects of discourse contain important information concerning the speaker's or listener's intent, tone, and attitude. The combination of speech impairments and the mask made it very difficult for me to interpret people's emotional states while conducting formal interviews. Occasionally, the man across the table from me would start crying without the usual warning signs of voice inflection and facial expression, causing me to suffer along with him from the knowledge that sometimes my best efforts to listen weren't good enough.

Studies of physician perception of PD patients with masking have found that the more severe the masking, the more negative are physicians' appraisals of PD sufferers' mood, cognitive ability, intelligence, and agreeability (Tickle-Degnen and Lyons 2004). Novice and experienced practitioners may differ, however, in their ability to draw upon other somatic clues for reading patient psychological or emotional states (Tickle-Degnen and Lyons 2004). My ability to rely upon other cues, such as body posture or movement, was useful for interpreting factual meaning, but I found them of lesser value when I was working to assess emotional meaning. In these instances I could sometimes rely upon caregiver commentary to inform me, but at times I found my limited skills to be an important reminder of how PD affects interpersonal relationships and communication. Even with my well-meaning efforts, I at times struggled to connect to the speaker's intended emotional world. Interactions with colleagues and other acquaintances must also suffer from their lack of effort and lack of ability to listen to the kinesics of PD sufferers' speech.

A Condition Affecting Feeling: Sadness, Depression, and Anxiety

Depression and anxiety are the most common psychiatric problems among PD patients (Dewey 2003; Schrag 2004). Depression is frequently found in the older adult population and is especially common among PD patients, with some estimates of prevalence as high as 40 percent (Friesen and Mateer 2001; Meara and Bhowmick 2000). Coincidence of depression and PD is bimodal; depression occurs most frequently in either the early or late stages. Whether this represents the difference between situational and endogenous depression is debated (Dewey 2003). Depression is often linked to low dopamine levels, implying a relationship with PD's underlying pathology (Dewey 2003; Fischer 1999; Meara and Bhowmick 2000). However, this does not translate into a dose-response relationship between PD severity and depression (Schrag 2004).

Neither depression nor anxiety is easy to diagnose in the context of PD. There is a considerable degree of overlap among these conditions (Schrag 2004). Hopelessness, pessimism, lack of motivation, and a desire to avoid social interaction may be attributable to PD's underlying pathology or to a coincident depression or anxiety (Dewey 2003). "Off periods," times when PD medications are not providing maximum symptomatic relief, may produce symptoms that are interpreted as depression, but that remit when medication efficacy is restored (Schrag 2004). Obviously, diagnosing depression or anxiety among PD sufferers is a complex endeavor, and the social stigma surrounding cognitive symptoms made it a difficult to broach the topic in interviews. Caregivers, more often than PD patients, shared with me descriptions of their partner's disabling anxiety or depression. Study participants tended to view depression as a sign of ingratitude and a moral failing; by admitting to having depression they were expressing a lack of appreciation for the abilities that still remained. As I learned more about how to broach the subject in the interview context, nesting it within a discussion of "How do you keep your spirits up?" or "The neurotransmitters involved in PD are also thought to be involved with depression; have you ever had any trouble with that?" I was able to tease out some discussion of psychiatric problems. While rather few sufferers would define PD as depression or anxiety themselves, it was evident that such symptoms dominated their lives.

Across the interviews, sufferers in particular who considered PD to be a condition of mood or anxiety described this experience in one of three general ways. The first was shaded by denial and emphasized the importance of comparing one's abilities to a worst-case scenario. Typical comments would describe how much worse off another PD sufferer was and emphasize how their own case was not too bad. For example, advising themselves to "accept it" and "don't give in," or explaining, "I'm not looking for pity," or "At least I've got my mind. Mrs. Smith's Parkinson's is terrible. She can't walk or eat. She doesn't even know her husband anymore. I can still get around okay"—all communicated that depression was something people considered, worked through, and experienced, even if it was not acceptable to discuss. The second response was to recognize that depression is an issue, but to downplay its significance. Such persons might describe a period of depression, but emphasize their recovery and locate depression squarely in the past. Most often they experienced these episodes early in the diagnosis and over time had assumedly come to terms with the prognosis. Finally, there was a small group of people who defined PD primarily as a condition affecting emotional life. Their experiences of depression and treatments underscore the somatic nature of both PD and depression. Invariably, this group identified the pathology of PD as the source of depression, and they viewed it as a biological condition appropriately treated with medication. As eighty-one-year-old Ralph describes it: "Well, first of all you have trouble slobbering. Then you have trouble being mobile. Then of course you have a tendency to be stiff. . . . You are not very well. You don't socialize too much with people. And the tremors. And depression goes along with Parkinson's. They walk hand in hand."

Fieldwork with depressed and anxious PD sufferers is challenging on many levels. Those who fell into the first category rarely discussed depression, and when they did it was in the limited context of another person's experience with it. What would be an appropriate response to someone who belittled another person's struggles with depression? Those who fell into the second category would hint that they had had depression, but when asked directly about it they would deny feeling depressed. Should I take this denial at face value? People who had lived through the Great Depression and fought in World War II may indeed not view these current limitations from PD as comparatively troubling. And how was I to regard those with obvious, untreated depression or anxiety, who were suffering but unable to recognize the course? What were my ethical obligations as a person and as an anthropologist? Had I possessed clinical training or operated under a mandatory reporting guideline, my role would have been clearer. But as an anthropologist and an outsider, it was often difficult for me to sort out my obligations in the context of sufferers' jokes about suicide or euthanasia.

Jokes about suicide and depression were the overarching themes of Henry's illness narrative. Henry's PD had taken away his ability to read, drive, and play golf—three key activities that framed his social engagement with and enjoyment of the world. The blows that his deteriorating vision and balance problems struck to his identity were compounded by more frequent memory lapses. Henry was an educator, an avid reader, and politically active. His inability to remember simple things like an old friend's name or even the day of the week was devastating to his sense of self. Henry, his wife, and I met one morning to talk about his life with PD. He was very friendly and we shared some laughs over politics (a subject I tended to avoid with the majority of participants). Later in the interview we discussed his PD and he was able to describe his earliest symptoms and the inkling he had that something was amiss, but his wife had to interject a timeline of events. I asked Henry to describe a typical day. He replied, "I take a lot of naps. . . . There are sometimes a week goes by and I don't get out of the house. If it's real cold weather I don't get out of the house." His wife noted that she strove to get him out of the house at least once a week, because she felt that social interaction benefited him. When I echoed her comments, he explained that it can be embarrassing, adding in a tentative, half-joking voice, "I don't know that I—I shouldn't say this, but I don't care that much about whether I get around or not. I'd about as soon take some pills that would get me over this. Got anything like that?" While Henry's motor symptoms caused him distress and limited his engagement with the world around him, it was the anhedonia that suffused our interactions that marked his experience of PD and aging.

Conditional Memory: Forgetting to Shake

Dementia is six times more likely in older adults with PD than those without and generally occurs later in the disease (Lang and Lozano 1998a; Rodnitzsky 2000). The risk factors for dementia coincident with PD include older age, longer disease duration, and moderate to severe motor involvement (Dewey 2003). However, PD dementia may be related to a co-existing AD (Woodruff-Pak 1997). AD and PD patients have similar types of plaques and tangles and researchers have hypothesized a relationship whereby AD and PD are located as two disease points along a continuum of somatic expression (Dewey 2003). The diagnostic challenge is to differentiate among AD patients who have parkinsonism, PD patients who also have AD, and PD patients with related dementia (Rodnitzsky 2000).

PD is associated with some short-term memory loss and a generalized slowing of cognitive processes (Fitzsimmons and Bunting 1993; Lang and Lozano 1998a). Sufferers also struggle with information retrieval, but dementia in PD affects executive function more than it affects language (Rodnitzsky 2000;

Friesen and Mateer 2001). Planning, initiation, regulation, and "goal-directed behaviors" are affected (Schrag 2004; Friesen and Mateer 2001). PD patients have trouble remembering how to perform basic motor scripts (Jankovic 2003). Thus, PD sufferers present with a variety of cognitive problems, from an inability to mentally sequence the steps involved in writing a check or getting out of a chair, to a limited ability to manage time and organize events, to difficulty recalling a specific word or name, to a slowing of mental processes. These sorts of memory loss are very distressing to PD sufferers, as they are unpredictable and inexplicable. Allen, an eighty-year-old PD sufferer, explains it this way:

> [My wife] will remember things better than I will, too. Whatever I say, believe what she says. Some of the tricks I pull, I went into the kitchen to take my medicine, I took my medicine out of the little container and set it on the shelf while I turned to get the water or something; I walked away and she found it later. I thought I had taken it when she found it. That's one of the things. Well, why didn't I remember it? It was right there and I was right there.

Whatever its ultimate cause, the onset of dementia is widely feared (Woodruff-Pak 1997), as this comment from Oscar, seventy-two, demonstrates.

SAMANTHA: How would you explain to someone what Parkinson's is?

OSCAR: That's one thing that I really can see. I call it a very individual disease, in that its different for everybody, in the symptoms and in the progression of it. I guess PD is a disease that you really have no control over. It's just a slow [process of]—but then that varies in progression—of losing your balance, losing your head. I've always been thinking too far ahead and I get concerned about what if I won't be able to drive. And I don't want anyone to have to take care of me. Like you see has already happened to some of our friends in the PD [support] group. [starts to cry]

As one man's comment about his PD diagnosis reveals—"At least it's not AD"—physical impairment is deemed preferable to mental. PD sufferers expressed pity for those who had both AD and PD and admired caregivers who stuck by their demented spouses, especially those who were able to care for their spouses at home. Study participants would joke that dementia is something to look forward to and there were several memory-related PD jokes in circulation, for example: "Researchers were prematurely excited about an experiment involving the administration of massive doses of vitamin E to a PD patient. His tremor, which had been severe, disappeared for about 90 percent of the time. Unfortunately it turned out that the poor patient had Alzheimer's, too, and was simply forgetting to shake." A few people casually mentioned that they would take their own lives or would rather die than develop dementia, and more than a few admitted that they worried about it. Forgetfulness was universally considered a sign of old age and the one thing that would "unmake" you. In this sense PD accelerated the destruction of the self and threatened one's individuality and integrity in ways more profound than mobility impairment did.

Impairments to executive can function occur in the presence or absence of dementia. I was interviewing Bonnie, a sixty-three-year-old woman who had had PD for more than ten years, at her farmhouse one hot summer afternoon. Bonnie does not have dementia but experiences other cognitive challenges. She had a few potentially dangerous instances of forgetfulness in which she forgot that she put something in the oven and only remembered six hours later when she returned to start dinner. She finds it difficult to attend to all of the details involved in organizing a family gathering. Choosing the date and time, orchestrating invitations, planning a menu, shopping for and preparing all the dishes, setting up tables and chairs, and ensuring that everything is completed at the appropriate time are now overwhelming activities. For many women, the decreased ability to plan had a negative impact on their roles as wife and mother (Solimeo 2008). Another woman shared her grief with me that she was no longer able to prepare large meals for her family. The basic mathematics of knowing when to start the roast, when to put the potatoes in, and when to make the rolls so that everything would be done at the same time was an inaccessible algebra. While Bonnie's fear of dementia led her to enroll in a memory aids course, others live with the uncertainty of whether the name that they couldn't recall was a symptom of the next stage. For these women, PD was lived as a condition that limited their ability to perform expected social roles.

Friends and family sometimes could not recognize the impact on sufferer's lives of conditional motor memory. Anthony, who at sixty-five years old had lived with PD for four years and was still working full-time, was frustrated at his brother's inability to understand the impact of his executive dysfunction. He said to me, "They don't understand the getting out of a chair. 'Is that all you got? You can't get out of a chair?'" His brother made light of Anthony's impairment, not realizing that it was not so much about the physical lack of strength to get up, but the mental process Anthony had to go through each time he wanted to stand. He had to think through each part of the movement. He placed both hands on the arms of the chair. He scooted himself forward. He leaned his weight over his knees—"nose over toes." He pushed up with his arms and moved slowly, so as not to fall forward. Once standing, he had to stay still for a moment to establish his balance. Anthony had to mentally walk through these steps in order to get up. He felt that he was an old man before his time: Sixty-five years old was old, but not that old.

Speaking on Condition: Communication Impairment in PD

Communication disorders are both biomechanical and cognitive. Speech is affected by tremor, memory loss, executive dysfunction, and anomia. PD sufferers experience reduced speech volume, uncoordinated articulation, and hoarse-ness. Their speech may become monotone, more rapid or slowed, slurred, or inaudible (Fitzsimmons and Bunting 1993). Virtually everyone that I encoun-tered has some degree of speech impairment, be it decreased speech volume, slurred speech, or a hoarse voice (see figure 3).

These changes pose problems in several areas. Many people had a difficult time using the telephone because the person on the other end could not make out what they were saying. This limited their ability to stay connected to lifelong friends and family. But perhaps the greatest problem speech impairment pre-sented was to interpersonal communication between married couples. The majority of study participants had lived in a rural area for most of their lives, and many of them had participated in agricultural activities that produced hearing loss. The combination of hearing loss and speech problem was aggra-vating. Anomia, the inability to connect words to objects, worsened this frustra-tion. I observed couples struggling with this tension in support group meetings and in the privacy of their homes. The PD sufferer would make a comment that their spouse could barely hear. The caregiver spouse would return the comment with a question. The comment would be repeated, but still at a level inaudible to the caregiver. On a few occasions I was privy to exchanges in which the care-giver interpreted their partner's inability to find the desired word as dementia or stupidity. These caregivers would repeatedly answer for their spouse or cor-rect their spouse's mischosen word. Sometimes this miscommunication was the source of arguments, and sometimes couples could laugh it off. As seventy-eight-year-old Ruby told me:

> I couldn't get the words to come out. . . . I noticed, just lately, when I am talking sometimes I feel like its not coming out. Like the words are stuck there or something. Like you can't say what you want to say. Then you get frustrated and that makes it worse. Like a simple word. Like for instance if I was trying to tell you, "The wind is blowing out there." I might forget what the word "wind" is. I'll say, "It's blowing out there." And he [her hus-band] will say, "The wind is blowing." He will tell me, you know. That's the frustrating part. You just can't get out what you want to get some-times. You talk softer. Like people with PD talk softer than they used to. I've noticed that, too. You can't get the words out; you kind of mumble or something. Then he [her husband] will say, "Speak up!" and I think, "Well, I was speaking up!"

While the fear of being trapped in the body, unable to communicate by speech was very real for a few of the people I met, a majority of PD sufferers live with a range of mild to moderate speech impairment. Several women explained that they had to drop out of the church choir or other social roles because they could no longer be heard. Men quietly bemoaned the loss of their strong, deep voices—a sign of masculinity and virility whose absence left them feeling like "little old men." Speech impairments, in a literal and figurative sense, robbed people of their voices. Men are supposed to have strong, deep voices, and PD sometimes reduced men's speech to a mumbled whisper. In contrast, women are expected to have soft voices; PD made their voices raspy, hoarse, and more masculine. An inability to communicate led sufferers to feel socially ostracized and shut out from longstanding social roles.

Speech (and hearing) problems presented an opportunity for participant observation in a way that I had not anticipated. By nature I am a soft-spoken person, and I had to practically shout in order to be understood by some older adults. I learned to speak more loudly, slowly, and directly. This process was an important way in which I gained perspective on communication problems in PD. While I often felt that I was shouting, to others my voice sounded as if it were at a normal volume. The exaggeration that I learned to normalize is similar to what many PD sufferers have to adopt, for both speech and affect. I honed my listening skills as well. As I listened for content to form follow-up questions, I simultaneously listened for the subtleties of inflection to compensate for the common lack of familiar body language. Most importantly, I became an interpreter, translating soft, hoarse, and mumbled Parkinsonian speech into discernible discourse. At one point, early on in my fieldwork, I called a male PD sufferer at home to set a date for an upcoming visit. When he answered the phone, I was unable to understand anything he said, as if he were speaking backwards and under water. I slowed my delivery down and increased the volume to where he could hear and understand my speech, but I was still unable to understand him. Frustrated with me, he handed the phone to his wife, who chastised him for answering it in the first place. She explained that not only did he have trouble speaking, but also he really wasn't making any sense, simply repeating words that he felt were what he wished to communicate but were to our reality simply a line of nonsense: "Apples, trucks, going to the store. Jane. Trousers." Her explanation assuaged my guilt a bit, but once again I was faced with my limited ability to honor another's personhood, limit their suffering, and finesse an uncomfortable social situation. Communication problems framed this man's condition on his social world, drawing it more tightly around him.

Parkinson's Is a Condition

The symptoms described here—tremor, depression, speech impairment, gait impairment, falling, the mask, forgetfulness, slowness, and executive function impairment—are not exhaustive of the range of physical problems reported by PD sufferers. What they represent are the symptoms that precipitated the most significant changes to individuals' sense of self and aging. PD can be defined as a percentage of the dopaminergic neurons that have died, as a syndrome, or as a neurological disorder diagnosed on the basis of three or four cardinal symptoms. Sufferers have heard these definitions from their doctors, self-help books, PD advocacy publications, and other media outlets, but even though many people are able to explain PD using medical terms such as "dopamine," "neurotransmitter," or "nerves," few people embody the disease in this way. As this chapter has shown, PD sufferers come to make sense of this disorder via the predominant somatic sign, and in doing so their articulation of how PD places conditions upon their lives reflects their notion of what it means to age.

When I asked people to explain what PD is, I was expecting to hear some variation on how PD is a neurological or nerve disease. I was not expecting that the question would provoke unease or anxiety. But this definitional question baldly raised the specter of PD's unpredictable and heterogeneous nature. Thus, when I asked people to explain to me what PD was, they would often start out by describing their symptoms and then connect these somatic experiences to their social experiences, and ultimately to their experience as an aging person. PD sufferers learn to incorporate biomedical terminology and explanations into their everyday discourse about PD, but they do not experience PD through them. When people used such terms as "dopamine" or "neurotransmitter," they did so to provide me what they felt was the correct answer, but such words did not reflect how they would describe it. Very few of the people I met would consider themselves to be anything but healthy people, and I was repeatedly assured that "I feel great, except for the PD." In this sense, for some people tremor is equated with PD and for others PD is equated with being slow. Across these somatic models, having PD means living with a condition that meaningfully alters one's identity. For Mildred, a seventy-year-old caregiver, "It's nasty. That's what I tell people. I think Parkinson's is really a nasty, hiding disease." Andrew, sixty-four, said: "I just have Parkinson's. And now, when you mention to somebody that you have Parkinson's, then they kind of shudder, sometimes. Well, I mean, some individuals would. And then sometimes I mention it and they say that they cannot see it in me."

SAMANTHA: How do you explain what PD is to somebody who doesn't know?

EDNA, SEVENTY-FOUR: Well, it's a progressive deterioration. That's about all it amounts to. Deterioration of your movements, your abilities to do things. It's old age. You don't know if it is or not.

SAMANTHA: How do you tell the difference?

EDNA: Look at Michael J. Fox. And he has a severe [case]; mine is called mild to moderate, I think. The medication hasn't changed in a long time. I do find myself slower. I'm slow. Then again, I'm old!

SAMANTHA: Is this what you thought it would feel like to be in your seventies?

EDNA: You know, I never gave it a thought. You don't feel like you have complete control of yourself. Of your life. You have to have your medication or you're going to get shaky. I guess I thought I'd live forever. And it ain't gonna happen! [laughs].

These comments, especially Edna's, show the disparate ways in which the condition of PD and the experience of aging intersect. Sufferers may follow the biomedical model in their compartmentalization of PD symptoms, but they do so not from the position of considering each symptom as if it were a separate and treatable disorder, but because they experience each symptom as a separate condition on their life, depending on their individual goals, expectations, and current age. Younger PD sufferers, age sixty to seventy, emphasized how PD symptoms sped up the process of social and somatic aging, making them feel old before their time. Sufferers in their seventies focused on the interplay of these conditions with normal aging and were more conflicted in assigning blame to one or the other process in constraining their life experiences. And the PD sufferers in their eighties and older emphasized how older age and normal aging was a greater condition on their lives than were individual PD symptoms. Thinking about PD as a condition on embodiment and how it comes to bear on the process of aging disrupts the script that PD and aging are both processes of inevitable loss and limitation. Rather, examining sufferers' definitions of PD as a set of unique conditions on their lives reiterates how both sickness and aging are products of the life course, wherever the cause may lie.

5

I Don't Know What to Blame It On

Introduction: Right Away We Thought of Insecticides

Edgar and his wife have lived in their modest home in a town of about five thousand people for the past forty years. They attend church weekly and a PD support group meeting monthly, as they are able. Every few weeks or so they get together with other family members to spend a day at a local casino or to share a meal at a local restaurant. Their children visit often and they enjoy being around their grandchildren. Edgar feels that his PD is pretty well controlled with a daily regimen of carbidopa-levodopa and ropinerole. He goes for physical therapy three times a week to help with his leg cramps and weakness, and he takes medications three times a day to treat his chronic obstructive pulmonary disease (COPD). To his mind, the PD doesn't bother him too much.

> The one thing that really irritates me is if I go to church, the first thing is that hand's going to start shaking. If we are at a place where we are going to be eating, you know, this hand is going to start shaking. It doesn't do it all of the time. That's what really gets to me is when that hand starts trembling. [It's embarrassing because] it's the one I eat with and it don't work too good. I cannot use my left hand. It just don't work.
>
> Sometimes, when I am working out there with wood I can't do what I want to do. If I am trying to get on that screw there, sometimes I don't get it on. . . . I do a lot of reading. I get books out of the library. I work on jigsaw puzzles quite a bit. . . . Well, you have to keep busy. You just can't sit around. The only problem I have, pretty much, is with the COPD. And if I take this [breathing] treatment here then I can go and do just about anything.

Now in his late seventies, Edgar was born in a rural section of a neighboring county. He met his wife at a country dance when they were in their late teens. After he served a year in the navy, they married and moved onto the farm. They have two children and several grandchildren, all of whom who live in Iowa. Edgar and his wife farmed for the first ten years of their marriage. They sold off the land, house, and implements and moved into a house in town when farming became too expensive and it was difficult to turn a profit. Edgar worked a few odd jobs here and there until he landed a position with a farm supply company. These operations typically sell farming implements, grain, and seed; build grain bins to order; and provide crop protection services, the application of pesticides and other agricultural chemicals. Edgar worked full-time for twenty-five years as a custom sprayer and metalworker, fabricating galvanized steel grain bins. About ten years ago he went to part-time work and for the past five years or so he has been keeping himself busy with his hobbies.

Edgar was seventy-two years old when one morning his hand started to shake as he was sitting at his kitchen table reading the morning paper. Over the course of a few weeks the shaking became so severe that his wife was finally able to convince him to see a doctor. Edgar told me he had no idea then what was wrong with him. His wife interjected, "I thought maybe he was doing something and that it triggered it or something. I thought it was just nerves. He's been a nervous person." The family doctor examined him, looking at his fingers and making him walk around the exam room. Edgar said, "When I walked down the hall, why, this arm was moving and this one wasn't. And [the doctor] said, 'That's PD. I know it's PD.' But I said that I wanted a second opinion."

A neurologist confirmed the diagnosis, and Edgar started to read more about the disease to see what might be in store for him. Edgar explained to me that the diagnosis per se didn't really worry him: "No, not really. It's there and it's always going to be there. So far, the medication, what I've been taking, has really got it controlled. The only problem I have once in a while is walking. I stumble a little bit while I am walking, which isn't too bad." But his wife added, "We were always wondering, How did he get this? That's what we were worried about most. And we right away thought [of] insecticides and all that."

Edgar's work with the farm supply company started out on a small scale. He would take a pickup truck out to the fields and apply chemicals with a ten-row sprayer. From there he graduated to a three-wheel sprayer with a sixty-foot boom. This is a much larger piece of equipment attached to a 4.5-liter diesel engine boasting a four-hundred-gallon spray tank. During the busy spring months Edgar ran it from five in the morning until ten at night. For about ten years, he ran this equipment from mid-March through July and in the fall was out in the fields again, spreading dry fertilizer. In the off times he worked installing grain bins and equipment, spending his days cutting galvanized steel and breathing in the acrid fumes.

I asked him, "Is that what you think it's from? The chemicals?" and he shared the following story with me.

That galvanized [metal] smoke is hard on you—it could be [involved] with
the PD, too. There's nobody in our family that's had PD. . . . I think it's
from the insecticides. I did get sick once. It was my own fault. I was supposed to take a couple of bags [of] pretty potent insecticide to a farmer
and it was raining a little bit. So what do you suppose I did? I put it in the
cab with me. When I got down there, I could start feeling it already. About
two hours later I couldn't go anymore. I couldn't maneuver [my body]. I
had a radio in the cab and so I called over to town and they come and got
me. I was out. It was from insecticide, for sure.

They took Edgar to the hospital for evaluation, but he was not admitted. "They
said it was fatigue. I know it wasn't fatigue. I had a splitting headache. It took me
two hours to get one pass around that field. I had to do something. There were
five or six or seven of them come out there to get me. When I said I was sick,
why, they got really worried."

Edgar hasn't said for sure whether he believes that this one incident is the
source of his PD, and he doesn't know of any other sprayers or metalworkers
who have PD. His wife explained, "I didn't think that he could ever have PD, you
know. We kept looking back at our families and no one had it." But Edgar added,
"It's there. It's always going to be here. Might as well live with it. Mmm. I get
along with it. I got to live with, so I get along with it."

Epidemiology and Local Knowledge

Scientific models for explaining PD incidence are incomplete and continually
changing. Neurological science and pharmacological developments have identified the brain's physiological malfunctions at increasingly minute locations,
and epidemiological evidence, though limited, demonstrates the relationships
among older age, exposure to potential neurotoxins, genetic susceptibility, and
PD incidence. Still, as with many disorders, medical science cannot yet explain
why one person with few risk factors for PD develops the condition while
another person who possesses multiple risk factors may never contract it. This
gap in the current theories undergoes contractions and expansions as knowledge of brain anatomy and function becomes more sophisticated, and it constitutes a place where social ideas about the aging process take prominence.

As a component of sufferers' explanatory model for PD, etiology emerged as
the sole place where the demarcation between aging and disease was straightforward, even if the cause of the disease was not. Treatment efficacy and mechanisms,
daily symptoms, disease presentation, symptom progression, and the diagnostic
process are all enmeshed in the tension between normal aging and disease. No one
ever reported to me that, after being diagnosed with PD, they believed that their PD
was a result of old age. PD sufferers learned about the various theories of disease

causation from the pamphlets that they picked up at their doctors' offices, from newspaper articles and television talk shows, from PD advocacy literature, and from their conversations with other people in the community or at support groups. They interpreted this information in light of their family history, occupational exposures, traumatic injuries, and other life experiences. The medical literature may not support sufferer-identified causes of PD, but they illustrate how people internalize and interpret such information, as well as how sufferers attribute blame for and come to terms with the diagnosis.

Scientific Perspectives on Parkinson's Prevalence and Incidence

PD may affect as much as 1 percent of the population over the age of fifty (Hopfensburger and Keller 1991), but assessing PD's prevalence is challenging. Many people living with PD have yet to be diagnosed, there is no public health surveillance of the disorder, diagnosed cases cannot easily be identified by medication use (not everyone is on the same medications and a minority do not take any medications), and the clinical definitions of what constitutes a valid PD diagnosis vary (see Rajput, Rajput, and Rajput 2003). Recent estimates for the United States indicate that at least 500,000 people are living with PD, with fifty thousand new cases diagnosed yearly (National Institute of Neurological Disorders and Stroke. 2000). An aging population contributes to projections that forecast a three- to fourfold increase over the next fifty years (Tanner and Ben-Shlomo 1999). PD is most predominant in white populations and lowest among Asian and black African populations (Lang and Lozano 1998a). Worldwide, the lowest PD rate is in China and the highest in Australia (Rajput, Rajput, and Rajput 2003).

PD incidence is hard to calculate because the disease develops slowly over time and people seek treatment at different levels of disability (Rajput, Rajput, and Rajput 2003). The most important predictor of PD incidence is age, and incidence differs more across age grades than by race or gender (Meara and Hobson 2000; Tanner and Ben-Shlomo 1999). The middle old (ages seventy-five to eighty-four) and oldest old (ages eighty-five and older) have the highest rates of PD (Berry and Murphy 1995). Nevertheless, epidemiologic differences in race, gender, and locality-based incidence may reflect poor reporting or underdiagnosed populations (Kirschstien 2000).

As with most chronic disorders, there are two major themes in the study of disease onset: genetics and environment. A family history of PD is a strong indicator of PD risk, and having a family member with PD increases the risk by two or three times (Lang and Lozano 1998a; Le Couteur et al. 1999). About one-fourth of persons with PD have an affected relative, but inherited, familial PD accounts for only 10 percent of all cases (Mizuno et al. 1999). Genetic inheritance is more closely linked to other parkinsonism variants than to idiopathic PD, and it is more strongly associated with younger onset, cases under the age of fifty (Farrer 2006). Seven genetic defects have been identified as causing parkinsonism, and about half of these are autosomally dominant Mendelian mechanisms, whereby having a single parent with the disease determines one's likelihood of developing it (Farrer 2006). Such findings may contribute to the development of diagnostic tools that could help identify preclinical cases or candidates for genetic therapy. Pinpointing a genetic substrate for PD may help researchers increase the power of epidemiological studies of environmental risk factors.

Views on the importance of environmental risk factors in PD etiology vary. Given the higher prevalence of PD among rural dwellers and men, a number of studies have explored the role of agricultural chemicals in PD incidence. These studies have examined classes of chemicals, dose, duration of exposure, and route of exposure. Studies examining the link between agriculture-related potential neurotoxins and PD have found either no increased risk or some increased risk (Kuopio et al. 1999). A meta-analysis of nineteen such studies determined that seventeen of them demonstrated a positive relationship between PD and pesticide exposure (Priyadarshi et al. 2000). A case-control study conducted in an urban area of the United States examined smoking, drug consumption, well-water use, exposure to heavy metals, and occupation, among other variables, and documented a slightly higher frequency of farming among PD cases (Wechsler et al. 1991). Koller and colleagues' (1990) study of 150 cases in Kansas evaluated their pesticide exposure, attending to its duration, route, and specific toxins. They found a statistically significant difference between cases and controls in the number of years of rural living, while Marder and colleagues' (1998) investigation of incidence among Hispanic, African American, and white elders found that having lived near a farm increased the risk of PD for African Americans but not for Hispanics or whites.

Internationally, results of case-control studies on agricultural exposures have produced conflicting results. Among a case-control sample in Finland, there was no statistically significant relationship between PD and potable-water source, or between involvement in agricultural work and PD (Kuopio et al. 1999). In Taiwan, where there is limited arable land and a high use of pesticides, a case-control study of PD patients and hospital controls determined that the risk of PD was greater among subjects who had used paraquat but could not identify a significant risk among occupational exposures to other potential neurotoxins (Liou et al. 1997). A thirteen-year cohort study conducted in Denmark found that agricultural and horticultural workers had a significantly higher risk of PD (Tuchsen and Jensen 2000). The French PAQUID cohort study examined the following risks for PD: occupational exposure to pesticides (including insecticides, herbicides, and fungicides), rural residency, and residency near vineyards. This work identified an increased risk of PD, AD, and low cognitive performance relative to occupational exposures, especially to fungicides (Baldi et al. 2003). The current understanding of the role of pesticides in PD can be summarized as this: The "weight of the evidence is sufficient to conclude that a generic association between pesticide exposure and PD exists, but it is not sufficient to conclude that this is a causal relationship or that such a relationship exists for any particular pesticide compound or combined exposure to pesticides and other exogenous toxicants" (Brown et al. 2006, 162).

Such mixed results are a product of the inherent complexities of PD epidemiology. Investigation into the causes of PD is limited by the inability to establish a temporal relationship between a specific environmental exposure and disease onset. Measuring the dose of an exposure is problematic as well. Exposures may be widespread and diffuse, such as a chemical found throughout the food or water supply. They may be direct and discrete, such as an identifiable physical contact with pesticides or mercury. Relevant exposures may occur over a long period of time, over a short period of time, or over a particularly vulnerable period of time (such as childhood). The route of exposure may be an important factor to consider (Le Couteur et al. 1999). Recall and survival biases intensify the challenge of epidemiologic investigation. For example, a seventy-year-old woman may not be able to recall the name of a pesticide that was used on the farm where she lived as a young girl. People who survive into late life may possess a special resilience or other characteristics that make them different from other people who had similar exposures or risk factors. Finally, epidemiologic studies of PD do not operate on a shared case definition (Le Couteur et al. 1999). Many researchers believe that PD arises from a complex combination of genetic predisposition and one or more environmental factors (Golbe et al. 1999; Vernon 1989).

An Embodied Etiology: Sufferers' Theories of Causation

To what do PD sufferers attribute their condition? PD symptoms and progression may overlap with what many elders see as normal aging, irrevocably changing sufferers' embodiment of aging as profoundly as it changes their physical and cognitive abilities, but PD sufferers don't believe that their disorder is necessarily a product of simple old age. At first, most people told me that they didn't know why they had it and—hopeful that I was privy to some new information—asked me if I knew what caused it. I ventured that there are a number of competing theories circulating throughout the scientific community and that no one really knows. When pressed to give my own opinion as to PD's source, I carefully presented a miniature literature review: There is a demonstrated association between some agricultural chemicals and PD; only a minority of PD cases can be tied to a genetic source. Given the ubiquity of agribusiness in Iowa and especially among the people with whom I worked, I expected that a number of people would associate their PD with agricultural chemicals. The notion that pesticides, herbicides, fungicides, or insecticides might cause PD was a volatile subject. Indeed, many PD sufferers and caregivers did raise such potential neurotoxins as a possible cause, but among *many* other possible PD triggers.

Figure 4 summarizes the diverse causes cited by the PD sufferers that I interviewed. A majority felt that agricultural chemicals, most often pesticides, could be linked to their particular case. Traumatic injuries, such as falls, broken bones, or head injuries, were the second most commonly cited source. A number of people discussed the possible ties between family history and PD, but there were equal numbers of people who reported a family history of PD and people who told me that it couldn't be genetic because they had no family with the disorder. Interestingly, the fourth most commonly mentioned cause was stress, almost always related to the death of a spouse. I could not identify any statistically significant relationships between the suspected PD trigger and the variables of current age, duration of disease, educational attainment, or self-reported fast- or slow-progressing cases. At first glance, gender appears to be the most significant factor, but this relationship is not significant when occupation is considered. While women and men both participate in productive, strenuous labor on the farm, no women in the study reported working directly with pesticides as salespeople or applicators. Only men discussed working with paints, solvents, galvanized metal, or welding, or reported having had carbon monoxide poisoning. On the farm or not, life in the country exposed almost everyone to potential neurotoxins associated with PD. But the meanings that sufferers attributed to such exposures were almost as heterogeneous as their disorders.

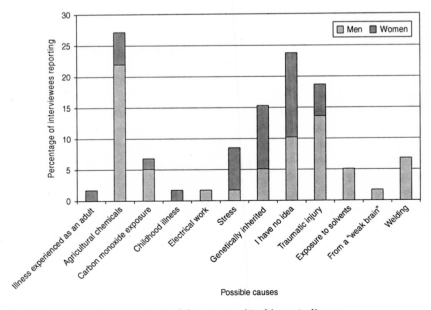

Possible causes

FIGURE 4 Interviewees' reports of the causes of Parkinson's disease

A Genetic Condition

When I asked people why they had PD, where it came from, about half brought up their family history. Joyce, seventy-five, told me, "They say that PD is not hereditary, but in our family my grandmother had it and also my mother. My brothers have essential tremors and also my sister has been diagnosed with essential tremors. It makes you wonder if there isn't some connection. My doctor tells me I'm the unlucky one with PD. My children are wondering what is ahead for them." More women than men referred to genetic causes, although the difference was not statistically significant. Respondents' understanding of how PD could be passed along through genetic material was a mixture of basic Mendelian mechanisms and folk models of inheritance. Some people believed that their PD could be inherited only if one of their parents had had it, whereas others believed that distant blood relatives such as a second cousin could contribute to an increased risk. Almost everyone who felt that their case was genetic had a first-degree relative with PD, but these cases were not always confirmed by diagnosis. Even though PD has been a diagnostic category for more than one hundred years, the generation of Americans who fought in World War I often did not live long enough to develop it, considered its symptoms part and parcel of old age, or were diagnosed with it prior to the 1960s advent of PD medications.

PD sufferers who believed their case to be genetically inherited thought back through family history and reconsidered their parents' behavior in a new light. Others knew firsthand the signs of PD in their parents or grandparents. One couple that I spent a good deal of time with both in and out of support group meetings determined that the wife's father's PD was the source for the wife's present case. The husband, Thomas, explained that "her dad had PD real bad. He wasn't able to do anything. He was so crippled up with everything that he couldn't talk or do anything. . . . Anna and I were in about our second year of retirement and I noticed that she started getting some of the same expressions that her dad had. I said something. He had so much trouble with the medication. They were giving him levodopa and every once in a while, about once a month, he'd just go out of his head. He'd take up a two-by-four and go through the door with it." Anna added, "Well, he could hardly walk. When he'd take off like that. We'd start looking for him close by and, heavens, he'd be clear up the hill in his pajamas. [laughs] Well, we talked about it. I agreed. I knew what my dad was like and I could see what I was doing was similar." I asked her, "What was that like, thinking about how your dad was and wondering if that was what you had?" She replied, "I think I handled it pretty good, even after they told me that I had it. I just did the best I could."

But the question, Will my children get it? remains, and the inverse, Because my father has it, should I expect it? emerges. One middle-aged bachelor, who managed to work full-time while caring for his disabled brother and his ninety-year-old father with PD, shared with me his concern. He subscribed to all the PD advocacy publications and tried to stay abreast of new research in the field. He did so in part to help his father but also to alleviate his underlying fear of developing PD himself. His brother's dementia and his father's PD increased his own risk for either condition. As he approached retirement age, he explained, the questioning was inevitable. With each new ache or pain he asked himself, "Is this a sign of PD?"

With his genetic heritage, he wondered what might be in store for him, but even when someone had a parent with probable or confirmed PD, they did not necessarily believe that genes were the cause. For example, Mary, a sixty-year-old PD sufferer, strongly believed that her case was related to pesticides, despite her mother having had probable PD.

> I think I know exactly how I got it. We lived in this house, which across the street had a field, either corn or beans, whatever. And the farmer was always spraying his produce. And one morning I woke up, and when I went to look out the window—we had twenty-two trees in our yard—and on most of the trees, all of the leaves on his side of the street had curled under. On half of the tree. I called the health department and whether they came out or not, I have no idea. But we never saw them come out. I thought that was really odd. Some kind of poison, really. So we lived for thirty years at that house. . . . I was exposed every day to that. See, my husband wasn't exposed as much because he went to work. You know, the kids would be around other places, they went to school and things like that. I was exposed more than anyone. And I believe that's it.
>
> But I also know, I think my mother might have had PD when she died. I didn't think about it at the time. Then one year she fell three times in our yard the summer before she died, and it didn't come together then. I didn't know I had PD then. When I look back on it, she was walking—we kidded her about walking like a duck. I think she had PD and we didn't know it. But I really believe that mine was from toxins.

Mary, despite mentioning her mother's case, linked PD to agricultural chemicals. Another woman, Helen, tied hers to a head injury she suffered as a young girl, even though she has two parents with PD. Because Helen's case emerged before those of her parents, she felt that genetics were not a factor: "It would be more like they caught it from me, wouldn't it?"

Working Conditions

Of all of the reported causes of PD, agricultural chemicals were the most common and contested. Edgar's exposure to pesticides, as described in the introduction to this chapter, was not unique. I was surprised and disturbed by the number of serious chemical exposures men in this group had experienced. In addition to residence in a rural area with possible exposure to agricultural chemicals in the air or in well water, participants described multiple instances of more direct contact with known toxins. They reported being sprayed by crop dusters, mixing pesticides by hand, and being doused with concentrated powdered pesticides. Protective equipment such as breathing masks, goggles, or plastic gloves were considered impractical or overly cautious, or were unavailable at the time, as these comments by PD sufferers Robert, seventy-four, then Jack, seventy-two, suggest.

> I read once that rotenone is thought to be one of the possible causes, and so if that's true that could be a source of some of my problem. Rotenone was an insecticide used on beef cattle. Beef have a parasite that gets into the stomach and then makes its way from the stomach out of the back of the cattle. We would buy the cattle from the range in the West, and you'd just run your hand across their back and they would have all of these little holes—little holes where the grubs were buried into the pelt of the animal. When cattle like that are butchered, their leather is just full of these little holes. To control them, we would use rotenone. And put it on pretty heavily and rub it in with our hands. And I am sure that we inhaled some of it, too. When we were on the farm, I guess for probably eight years, I showed beef at the county fair and would have been working some with that insecticide during that time. . . . Well, on the farm we used herbicides also. Spray. We never were as cautious as we should have been, probably. It's the farmwork. We didn't use the real powerful herbicides that are used today, but we did use the insecticides.

> Another thing it could be: We worked with fifteen or twenty chemicals down there at [the dairy plant]. Nobody explained to you the dos or don'ts about the chemicals. . . . You never had gloves. You never had goggles. You never had a respirator. Every once in a while some idiot would mix chlorine and rinse it out and it would make chlorine gas immediately. You'd better be out of there, because you are not going to last fifteen minutes in there. . . . That might have been where it come from, I don't know. . . . They used to put you in a tanker to scrub it out by hand. You were in there with the damned stinking chemicals. They had one guy, they finally went looking for him, and here he was lying in the tanker. The paramedics said if he had been in there another five minutes, we wouldn't have had to call. He had a lot of lung problems. He finally died of cancer of the lung.

The attribution of blame to agricultural and other chemicals depends on people's relationship to them. Men who worked for chemical companies or in private industry, either delivering or spraying farm chemicals or using them daily as part of their job, were more likely to be openly critical of their exposures. Men who applied chemicals that they purchased for their own farms were less likely to attribute PD to that exposure. When the subject of agricultural chemical usage on their own properties arose, with a few exceptions, they were quick to present one of several arguments. They explained that the chemicals that they used on the farm could not have caused their PD because otherwise their wives would also have it. Another argument, as Bonnie mentions, denies that overuse of agricultural chemicals could be the culprit because they cost too much.

Bonnie and her husband have lived on and operated a medium-sized farm of about three hundred acres since they married more than thirty years ago. At sixty-three, Bonnie traces her PD back to a particularly strong reaction to the insecticides that they applied to their crops but was reluctant to fully blame chemicals for her condition. When I asked her to share her thoughts on the cause of her PD, she explained:

> I don't know. I am beginning to think that it was chemicals. But I had to have the right cells or physical makeup to be susceptible to it, because my husband and I were both in the same field that day that I suspect maybe [caused my particular case]. We talk about it; we have now gone and pinpointed the day and the year that that happened. I just felt ill. I was rotary hoeing. I don't know if you know what rotary hoeing is, but you pull it and it has a wheel with tines on them. You drive fairly fast through the fields. It would flip out the weeds, but not the corn or beans. I was doing that and they had sprayed the field. And my husband was cultivating, where they go through with shovels and they tear out any weeds that are in between the rows. And so we were both in that field that day. I just got to feeling not well. I said, "I am going to the house." I took the tractor home and I laid down and I just felt nauseous. By that evening or the next day I had laryngitis, and it lasted three weeks. And I never [before] got laryngitis or anything. I could not talk on the telephone, because I could not be heard. I didn't think a lot about it. It just went on and then finally it went away. I have often wondered if that day was somehow the beginning of it.
>
> My husband was very defensive when we first had the diagnosis of PD and they talked about it being chemically related. And people on the farm. And he is very defensive about the chemicals and things we use on the farm, because we don't overuse them. For one thing, they are expensive and we don't want to! [laughs] Like [he] said, "The rate that people use them on their yards, of some of the chemicals, are far greater ratio than what we use on the farm." But we haven't pushed it. It's like, what difference does it make? But, I'd kind of like to know. I am sure we will sometime. . . . I guess I would like to know some origin of it.

The argument against pesticides as a potential cause is an economic one. Farmers argue that, because they were so costly, agricultural chemicals were used carefully and sparingly.

A Nervous Condition: Stress, Nerves, Trauma, and PD

Stress and traumatic injuries are one area in which gender emerged as a significant variable in the attribution of blame for PD. While both genders are represented in these categories, as causes of PD, women were more likely to bring up stressful life circumstances, and men were more likely to identify a traumatic injury or illness. Among men, such injuries included broken bones and other hospitalizations. These incidents served as important markers of disease onset. Henry, now eighty-two years old, believed that his long convalescence from influenza wreaked havoc on his body and allowed the PD to emerge. Everett broke his wrist playing tennis one spring and noticed a tremor in his arm a few weeks later. At first he thought that the tremor was a side effect of the fracture—that perhaps the break had somehow caused nerve damage to that arm. Another man fell off a ladder and broke his ankle. After his eight-week recovery he noticed that he had a tremor in one side and that he felt "shaky" all the time. He explained that his fall must have "shaken something loose" that started the PD. These men connected the tremor to something internal that loosened up whatever it was that causes PD in the brain, leading to its emergence in the body.

Two women mentioned concussions as a possible source of PD, but a majority of women in these categories mentioned stress as the culprit. Stress was most often a result of the death of a spouse or long-term illness in the family, as in Jeanne's case. Jeanne is sixty-seven years old and has had PD for about six years. She retired at sixty-two and feels that her PD is due to stress, even though her aunt died from PD and her mother may have had it. She explained, "It was just stress. And I really believe that stress does a lot of things to your body." Jeanne went through a long period of major life changes and stressful events. She took care of her husband at home for five years up until his death nine years ago.

> He had pulmonary fibrosis and cancer. He went from [weighing] about 210 to about 90 pounds. And he couldn't breathe. He just kind of drowned. . . . He went into the hospital for a heart check. The doctor said that his heart was okay, but he sent him to the hospital for a biopsy. It was a minor surgery. They did the biopsy, but on the table he had heart problems and they had to do a pacemaker real quick and then he got staph [infection]. He was sick and was in intensive care for almost two months, if you can imagine. That man went through hell. They put him on an antibiotic and he reacted badly to the antibiotic and it destroyed his clotting mechanism. They had a swan catheter in him and they had an arterial line and they had to pull all of those things out. They had to cauterize him. They had to stop the bleeding.

Her husband stayed in the ICU for three months, was readmitted the following year for another extended stay, and then was released to die at home. As Jeanne explained, "He didn't want to go back into the hospital, but I couldn't control him anymore. He was lacking oxygen and so he was fighting everything and trying to walk, but not being able to. It was really bad."

Jeanne was able to work part-time while caring for her husband, but then she suffered a devastating burn that contributed to her early retirement. Jeanne found the incident painful and stressful, and she felt that the process of seeking care was more than she could handle.

> [My hand] was just black from the flames. I threw the oil out and came back in and put it under cold water right away. And then I got in the car and I drove to the doctor's office. And they looked at it and said that it was burnt too bad for him to do anything and that I had to go over to the burn clinic. . . .
>
> The stress of it—it was just very emotional for me. In fact, I think stress caused my PD. Because I had just taken care of my husband and lost him and then to burn my hand. I was very stressed out with that burned hand. It took a long time to heal. It took a very long time. I really didn't care to ever go into the hospital again. Isn't that crazy? I just didn't want to work anymore, and I loved nursing. I am so happy retired. I love it. But I knew my last year at work that I was having some problems with PD. I kind of diagnosed myself. I knew as a nurse, but I never wanted to admit it.

In spite of her nursing background, Jeanne connected her case to life events rather than to biomedically accepted theories. The idea that emotional stress could cause the PD to emerge was explained to me by another woman, Ruby, seventy-eight when we talked, who went through multiple emotional hardships with her family. Ruby's son-in-law suffered from leukemia and then later fell off a third-story scaffolding. At the same time one of her sons was arrested on a drug charge and later incarcerated for several years. She was trying to manage these various family crises while suffering from an overwhelming sense of fatigue and depression. Her hands started to shake while she was attending the six-week trial for her son, and she sought her doctor's advice.

> After that, then they finally diagnosed me. I felt like, kind of like a load was being lifted from my shoulders. You think you are going nuts. [laughs] Nobody knows what is the matter with you. You know there's something the matter, but you don't know what it is. . . . They just kept telling me that I was in a state of depression, you know. Well I was. I did a lot of crying. It was a relief when they finally told me that I had PD. I knew then I wasn't losing my mind. I thought something was terribly [wrong]; I guess I was relieved to find out that there was something, that it wasn't in my mind. I was also very thankful that they didn't tell me that it was AD. . . . I really don't know, but I've always said it was stress, because I've had a very stressful time.

Ruby explained to me that these stressful life events made her nervous and that stress affects the nerves. She thought that "nervousness" led to the shaking and started the PD process.

A Puzzling Condition

Even people with several potential risk factors did not always identify a single cause for their case. Lawrence, eighty-one, relates that "we have tried to figure out what I could have done. I have been hit in the head hard. I used to work at a moving and storage company and they warehoused chemicals. We used to unload cartons and sacks of copper sulfate. I would always get sick when we'd do that. It would make me nauseous and dizzy. I thought maybe that contributed to it. I have not the slightest idea. We have always tried to figure stuff out." Almost one quarter of interviewees had no theory for why they developed PD (see figure 4). Among those who had virtually none of the risk factors save older age, the topic of "clean living" emerged. As one avowedly clean liver, Edna, seventy-three, explained, "It's not in the family. It can't be inherited, because nobody had it that I know of. . . . Never drank any liquor to speak of, never smoked. What did that one doctor say? He said that it seems like it hits people that are nice people. I don't drink coffee, I don't smoke, and I've never had a beer. He said, 'You nice people are paying a price!' " She laughed.

The literature on PD risk factors supports Edna's assertion. Several epidemiological studies have demonstrated the protective effects of caffeine and nicotine for PD, but they stop short of recommending such behaviors for disease prevention. Self-described clean livers puzzled over what might have caused their PD and then eventually came to an understanding that it didn't matter why they had it. The goal now was to accept it and move on with life.

Another way in which people dealt with the puzzling question, Why me? was that PD was a condition related to the age we live in. In many ways, they are right. The prevalence of PD is increasing, even when rates are adjusted for age. This increase may be due in part to improved diagnostic criteria or earlier detection, but many PD sufferers believe that there is a true increase in cases because of the number of chemicals people are exposed to at work and over the course of their lives. While there were few statistical associations among gender, age of onset, current age, and sufferer-identified causes of PD, it is clear that lay understandings of etiology internalize biomedical and epidemiological theories and interpret them in the context of their own life experiences.

PD is likely not a normal or inevitable consequence of greater age, and PD patients separate the causes of PD from the biological aging process. Yet this is where the salience ends. The distinction of the disease from normal aging provides people with a way to come to terms with the disorder and to enact a degree of separation from their own bodies. This separation, while predominantly based on neurological models of the disorder, functions to support elders' experience of growing older. While PD is currently incurable, the fact that it is a disease caused by something other than aging gives people hope. They come to accept it as a condition of and affecting life, but even as they speak about accepting the diagnosis and moving on with life, they orient themselves towards fighting it as a discrete entity distinct from their body. The rationales that sufferers create for the cause of PD help give meaning to their disordering condition. As PD symptoms conspire with their own aging bodies to transform retirement into a period of accelerated losses, confusion, or disavowal, linking PD to something outside their control such as a pesticide exposure or genetic inheritance gives them something to hold onto. And for those who have "no idea" why they are "the lucky ones" with PD, the not knowing can be just as meaningful, working to move them past the wondering and toward the practicalities of negotiating a life with shaking hands.

An Unpredictable Condition

Chronic conditions are multifactoral and products of lifelong genetic, behavioral, and environmental factors. Just as sufferers come to the diagnostic encounter expecting that their unknowing will be resolved, they address the question, Where did this come from? with a similar hope for resolution. In both cases, PD sufferers are presented with a huge amount of data that has yet to yield definitive answers. Sufferers then seek to make sense of their condition in the context of their own lives, interpreting their experiences and exposures through a filter of biomedical theories. Yet, despite their integration of largely scientific explanations, their attribution of blame is intrinsically related to who they are and their social relationships to the causative agents.

For sufferers who determine a genetic predisposition to PD, the blame game is straightforward and there are no guilty parties. No sufferers felt that their parents or grandparents were to blame for causing their current case of PD, but they did often wonder if they had unwittingly passed along a gene to or increased the likelihood of the disease for their children. And adult children of PD suffers questioned their own somatic experiences in light of the increased possibility that they, too, could develop PD. In this sense, PD as a genetic condition certainly cast a shadow over the experience of growing older. PD sufferers who linked their case to chemical exposures seemed to do so only if they were not personally and directly at fault for misusing such substances. Yet they were generally reluctant to go so far as to blame their former employers for not protecting them from risk. What would you say to such men or women, whom you've known for thirty years, who attend the same church, and who have health concerns of their own? And if it's their fault, then why hasn't everyone who worked for them developed PD? The self-reliance and independence of rural Iowans underlie these discussions, as individuals take responsibility for their own health; some sufferers believe that a preoccupation with the root cause of the PD is a sign of ingratitude for those abilities they still possess.

Interestingly, regardless of whether sufferers had a single theory for why they developed PD or had adopted a multicausal view, no one attributed their PD solely to growing older. PD and aging come to be experienced coincidentally, with one condition informing and influencing the other in an inextricable relationship. I asked Lawrence, who was eighty-one, why he thought he had PD. "That, I don't have the slightest idea," he said. "The pope has had it. The boxers have had it. Michael J. Fox has it. But I don't know why or what you have to do to not get PD. I have lived a pretty clean life and I can't really understand why this tremor came. I don't think anybody does yet. I have thought about that: Why did it happen to me? What did I do? But it happened and you just accept it and go on. . . . PD is a disability, all right. Of course, when you get to my age, you don't know if it's PD or old age that's getting you." PD may be a condition, but like many conditions, it is something that this generation of elders accepts and learns to live with.

6

I Don't Know What's Worse, Parkinson's or the Medications

Introduction: After a While They Start to Get You and They Don't Let Go

Gordon and Irene, both now in their early seventies, had met and married in their early twenties. They raised four children and have three grandchildren, all of whom live within a day's drive. Irene worked at home, taking care of the children, and spent time volunteering at the county library. Gordon worked as a lineman for the local electric company—"a rather dangerous job," as he put it—for forty years. They lived in the same house for more than forty-five years and have always resided within ten miles of their birthplaces. Gordon had looked forward to a retirement packed with fishing and hunting trips and more time to spend with his family. PD has drastically altered their anticipation of the golden years.

Gordon was working full-time and not yet anticipating retirement when his PD symptoms first appeared. Thinking it was just "nerves," his employer moved him to successively less demanding positions, but to no avail. Gordon's tremor became more pronounced and disabling, and he became unable to perform even the most basic responsibilities, such as driving around to check on job sites. He retired on Social Security Disability Income in his midfifties. Shortly thereafter Gordon was in the hospital having heart-valve replacement surgery and the cardiologist recognized his shaking as something other than nerves. He was referred to a neurologist, who diagnosed him with PD. He had been having symptoms for more than two years.

Irene had to adjust to having Gordon at home all the time. After having organized her days around her own interests and volunteer activities, she recognized that she now needed to shift the focus of her life from her schedule to the demands of Gordon's condition. His PD symptoms became more severe, and he began to have trouble putting words together. Given enough time, he would speak, but his speech became slower and softer. Gordon became more unsteady on his feet and increasingly prone to falling. Irene gradually adopted more and more of their household's decision-making power and finally decided that they had to relocate to a more accessible apartment. Thinking ahead, she wanted to divest herself of home ownership in case they had to move Gordon to a long-term care center. Irene sold their home and moved them to an apartment, which they rent on a month-to-month basis. Over time, the stress of caring for Gordon led Irene to place him in an adult day-care center part time. She explained that she could no longer leave him at home alone and she needed time to manage household duties, as well as some time to herself.

Even with Gordon in day care, Irene was worried about him:

> Gordon is unusual, as the day-care [staff] says, because sometimes he's real good mentally and sometimes he's terrible. Usually, when he's real stiff, I think his brain slows down, too. When he's bad physically, he's bad mentally. And not many people are like that. Most of the people they deal with are one thing or the other. He said he was only going outside to get a breath of air, but she told me that last week he tried to get out the back door again. And she said, "You see, we trust him, because most of the time he is fine." But then, when he isn't, that's bad. They stopped him, but he did get away two times. He knows well enough when they are busy. . . . He had been imagining things happening at [day care] that weren't at all, you know. But, they were real to him and he thought that he just had to get away from it, didn't you?

Gordon added, "I can run faster than average."

A sense of frustration and of that eerie stillness before a storm engulfed me when I met with Irene and Gordon for an interview one afternoon. Irene recounted Gordon's history of PD, pausing from time to time to give him an opportunity to join the conversation. We discussed their recent relocation, the day care, and Gordon's complex medication regimen. While Gordon viewed his PD symptoms as major barriers to living the retired life he had imagined, Irene felt that his real problem was not the PD per se, but all the medications.

IRENE: They started him on mirtazapine first, and it made him as crazy as a hoot owl on that. Then when I told them, they switched him to paroxetine HCl, and that has been a little better. I never did see any side effects from that. I don't know if he's depressed [now]; I think he was then. He cried a lot. He hasn't done that since he's been on paroxetine HCL.

You know, the side effects of the pills are almost worse than the disease. You've heard that before, I suppose. I think that people who are new on it, they think the pills are great—once they get on carbidopa-levodopa and they can move. And he did the same thing. Then after a while they start to get you and they don't let go. It's hard. It's a real problem.

[The doctor] says that, given a certain number of days [without medication], he'd lay in bed like a rock and wouldn't be able to move. Well, we can't hardly have that. So then he takes all of these pills—nine kinds, between heart and PD, you know. The two kinds of carbidopa-levodopa—he takes a low dose of the quick release in the morning and then the rest of the day it's continued release. He's also on pramipexole dihydrochloride. He used to be on other PD drugs, but one by one they cut those out as useless. Like tolcapone. And some others. He took all of those drugs that are supposed to help the carbidopa-levodopa. He started on that first one, bromocriptine. And then he was on pergolide mesylate, something else, too.

I can vouch for the strength of them. I took his pills one night by mistake. I was on the phone and I had my pills and my water there and I was going to give him his. It was late. As soon as I did it, I knew [that I had taken his pills by mistake]. I hallucinated during the night. I did. It was just as clear [as day]. . . . I swore that I saw a whole bunch of bees and wasps against the ceiling. I couldn't have. The room was dark, for one thing. Part of me was sane enough to know that. I told myself, "You didn't see those. It's dark in here. You couldn't." But that was one pill. I mean, that was one dose. And he has probably had thousands and thousand of doses, with residual effect. And [the doctor] can't raise the drug level. Gordon takes too much as it is, you know. See, he doesn't realize that [he hallucinates]. [Speaking to Gordon] Although you know that you probably do, because everyone tells you that you do.

GORDON: That I do what?

IRENE: Hallucinate. See things that aren't there. Every day, at least. Frequently, you see things that aren't there. He really sees it, so he can't believe me that it isn't there. [laughs] Of course, I look and I just see what is really there. Sometimes I just walk away, because I don't want to fight over it. He does see it. His mind creates that for him. And it's all those pills, I'm sure.

[Last year] Gordon thought people were following us in cars and trying to hurt us and things, peering in [to our apartment]. Anyhow, when I wasn't home one time he called 911 because [he thought that] they were gassing him in the apartment. The doctor in the emergency room [admitted him for treatment and came to speak with me.] I said, "You know, I know he does that. We are handling it." And he said, "Lady, when somebody calls 911 and says that somebody's gassing them, you are not handling it. He has to see a psychiatrist." So ever since he's gone to see the psychiatrist. And it really hasn't made a whole lot of difference, either.

After Irene related all this to me, she left the room for a bit to give Gordon greater incentive to talk. Gordon and I spoke about the things he would do if his "thinking were better," as he put it, and his tremor not so disabling. He would take long drives in the country. He would wake early to go fishing in his rowboat. He would not be attending the adult day care, which he did only grudgingly. I asked him if he found anything in particular frustrating about his disability. He replied, "Probably the worst thing is that I abuse Irene. Not physically—she's a good talker and I am not. I am with certain things. I can't even tell you. But I start to shake and it's hard to calm myself down. I sometimes think I am seeing people looking at us. Like [in] this apartment. I don't know what else to say about it." We both fell silent for a bit, enjoying each other's company, but at the same time there was a shared acknowledgment of impending loss. For that time, as we sat there looking at each other, we recognized that his PD was only going to get worse, that his abilities were deteriorating, and that there was nothing to be done. Even though it was not my role to heal Gordon's body or life, I felt powerfully ineffectual. But Gordon didn't seem to hold me accountable for my limitations. He felt badly for putting his doctors in the position of not being able to do their work. That quiet time together was a moment of shared grief and camaraderie.

Irene came back into the room and we began to wrap up our interview.

IRENE: The mornings are his best time. He actually reads the paper in the morning, don't you? Usually in the evening he will look at books and the paper, but he isn't really reading. He goes over and over the same page. But in the morning he reads the paper, because if I ask about something, he knows what it was that was in there. Mornings are his best time, and as the day goes on it gets worse. He sleeps most of the time, don't you?

GORDON: Yep.

IRENE: Just sits in the chair and sleeps after supper. We like different things, don't we?

GORDON: [To me] Can you see?

SAMANTHA: The pictures over there?

GORDON: No, past them. You have got to be down about here.

SAMANTHA: [I move over to where he is seated and crouch down next to him.] Yes?

GORDON: What do you see?

SAMANTHA: Past the pictures? I see the hallway.

IRENE: And the bedroom and the window. What do you see out the window?

GORDON: [To Irene] Shhh. Not your turn. Okay. Let's try that again. What do you see near the top of that open frame there? Do you see a pole?

SAMANTHA: I see a pole outside.

GORDON: There's a pole out there. It's a—what do they call that? The crisscross all the way up? It's a lattice-type pole. It's steel.

SAMANTHA: I see that.

GORDON: Near the top of the light there is a man on that pole.

SAMANTHA: There is?

GORDON: There is. In my estimation.

SAMANTHA: What's he doing?

GORDON: Well, he's working up there. He's either putting up lights or—[Gordon gets up and walks toward the window. I stand up to follow him.]

For a time I had no idea what was going to happen. Would Gordon become combative, as had one man who threw a notebook across the room and stormed out of his apartment, midinterview? Would he become adamant and argumentative, including me in his list of people out to persecute him? Or would he start weeping, something that I had rarely witnessed prior to fieldwork—grown men overcome with emotion sobbing for both what had been lost and what remained to be taken away? Those moments of not knowing were a glimpse into the kind of uneasy uncertainty with which many PD sufferers continuously live. Gordon turned to me, shoulders slumped, eyes vacant and lost. Crestfallen and sheepish he said, "Oh, he's gone now." I imagined that the man on the pole was Gordon, living out the life he expected. Gordon was out there on the electrical pole, still working and physically fit, but now recognizable only to himself, and fleetingly so.

Therapeutic Relief

It is important to note that there are no cures for any of the major neurodegenerative diseases. In the case of PD, there are a number of pharmacologic and surgical approaches to reducing the severity of PD symptoms. Prescription medications are the primary therapy, and virtually all PD sufferers will take at least one to alleviate their symptoms. Prescription medicines have the benefit of being a familiar intervention, of being amenable to the individualized regimen that each sufferer requires, of being economically accessible (to a degree), and of being noninvasive and reversible. However, prescription medicines' cost, issues pertaining to polypharmacy and comorbidity in later life, the complexities of adherence and administration, side effects, and their inability to adequately control late-stage PD make them imperfect therapies. For severe PD cases, surgical interventions may present a compelling advantage. Pallidotomy and thalamotomy—surgeries in which the affected portion of the brain is deactivated—and deep brain stimulation can dramatically improve some nonresponsive or intractable cases. However, the high cost and the invasive, risky, and irreversible nature of such surgeries makes them a choice of last resort. And many neurosurgery clinics may limit eligibility to PD sufferers under age seventy. Complementary and alternative medicines, physical therapy, chiropractic, and speech therapy coexist as adjunctive therapies—never replacing medicines but often filling in the gaps in medication efficacy, such as chronic pain and rehabilitation.

Prescriptions

At the time of my fieldwork, there were several types of drug therapies in use—anticholinergics, dopaminergics, and dopamine receptor agonists (DAs) (Fitzsimmons and Bunting 1993). The carbidopa-levodopa patch, apomorphine injection, and rotigotine patch had not yet received FDA approval. Anticholinergics treat tremor and the effects of slowness by blocking acetylcholine receptors, thus increasing the relative level of dopamine in the brain. Dopaminergic medications (namely carbidopa-levodopa) treat rigidity, slowness, and tremor. These medications are precursors to dopamine that the body converts to dopamine in the brain. They are generally combined with another drug to ease nausea or to increase dose longevity. Almost all older PD sufferers take carbidopa-levodopa, extended release carbidopa-levodopa, or carbidopa-levodopa plus entacapone. DAs primarily control motor fluctuations.

In addition to these three kinds of medications, PD patients are likely to be taking drugs to address carbidopa-levodopa side effects or particularly recalcitrant PD symptoms, to lengthen the efficacy of levodopa, or to treat another underlying condition. Such medications may include antidepressants, laxatives, antipsychotics, anti-inflammatories, osteoporosis medications, high blood pressure and heart medications, or pain medications. Over-the-counter vitamins were also used by many participants, both at the recommendation of a physician and because of patient-held beliefs regarding the ability of specific vitamins to slow PD progression or alleviate symptoms.

Participants described their medication history in the context of their illness narratives, and in support group meetings many conversations revolved around the subject of medications. Across all these sites, medications were framed as both blessings and banes. Medication management is an individualized affair, and it often takes months to arrive at the right dose and combination. This process left many people with a collection of half-used prescriptions; an established regimen may last only a year, as disease progression warrants changes on its own calendar. Although support group members redistributed some of these medicines, many went unused, sitting in kitchen cabinets as expensive reminders of failed therapeutic responses. The lengthy trial-and-error phase, the sight of wasted medicines, and the specter of the shoebox full of pill bottles on the kitchen table made many people feel like "guinea pigs."

Sufferers are right to label themselves as such, for experimentation is the rule rather than the exception. From onset of treatment, medications are used to validate the diagnosis and to alleviate symptoms. Unfortunately, despite clinical algorithms designed to simplify PD pharmacotherapy, it can be hard to predict a patient's response to medicines. All the PD medications cause side effects, especially carbidopa-levodopa, which produces the embarrassing and frustrating uncontrollable movements called dyskinesias. Some of the dopamine receptor agonists caused alarming hallucinations or psychoses. The lore of the "medication honeymoon" circulated among support groups: Sufferers are delighted by the efficacy of medications at the onset of their condition and then dismayed to learn that carbidopa-levodopa may be effective in treating symptoms for only seven to ten years. After that honeymoon, the balance between effective dose and medication side effects favors adverse effects. At every support group meeting I listened to at least one conversation about the limitations of medicines, from the lack of a pharmacological cure for PD, to the frustration at having to take one medication to alleviate the side effects of another, to their incomplete and transitory efficacy and their economic burden.

Medication use and reporting varied widely among participants. I asked questionnaire respondents to check off their current PD medications, estimate their monthly out-of-pocket medication expenditure, and describe their health insurance coverage. While a handful of PD sufferers in the study took no medications (5 percent), almost 60 percent of questionnaire respondents took three to five PD medications, along with medications for other conditions (see figure 5). PD medicines were taken at a considerable cost, with a monthly average out-of-pocket expense of $161. A number of men were able to obtain their medicines at no or low cost ($7 per medication) from the Veteran's Administration, but half of all respondents paid between $10 and $2,500 per month out of pocket.

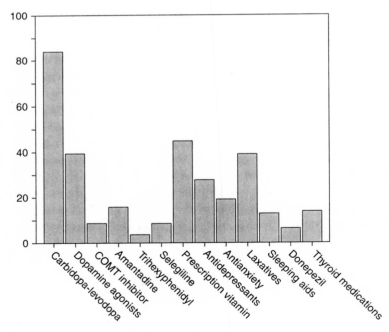

FIGURE 5 Percentage of questionnaire respondents reporting use of specific prescription PD medications

Most PD sufferers explained that they had never been "pill poppers." The knowledge that they had to take a medication every day for the rest of their lives, and that without it they would be unable to function, was at times a depressing and onerous weight. This cohort of elders who had lived through the Great Depression and World War II was used to toughing it out, and many were not the type to "run off to the doctor for every little thing," as one man explained to me. And yet they were disappointed to start carbidopa-levodopa and find that it didn't completely restore them to full functioning. While some people were deeply grateful for the relief, others were frustrated to have to take several medicines that only partly improved their function. And others, as eighty-two-year-old Henry assured me, took their medicines to no discernible effect.

SAMANTHA: For the PD, right now you are on the carbidopa-levodopa, donepezil HCL, the quetiapine fumarate, and the vitamin E. And you don't feel like they are doing anything for you?

HENRY: I can't see that they do.

SAMANTHA: So why do you keep taking them?

HENRY: That's a good question. [laughs] I guess I don't have the guts enough not to take them.

Carbidopa-Levodopa: From Medication Honeymoon to Medication Window

Although seven new drugs were approved for the treatment of PD in 1997 alone, carbidopa-levodopa remains the preferred treatment (Fischer 1999; Lang and Lozano 1998b). Discovered in 1908, levodopa is a dopaminergic compound used to restore motor function. It does not slow disease progression. There tends to be a dramatic initial improvement from the medication, but over the long term the medication's efficacy lessens and its side effects increase (Iansek 1999; Wallhagan and Brod 1997). Because of the lifespan of the medication's effectiveness, there is some debate on when during the disease progression it is best to start prescribing it. Up until the past decade, PD sufferers were often prescribed comparatively high doses in an effort to resolve all motor symptoms and restore normal appearance and function. Now it is more common for neurologists to advise patients to delay initiating this medication and to take as low a dose as possible until their symptoms become too burdensome. Sufferers try to find a happy medium between embarrassing and limiting symptoms resulting from too low a dose and a relatively symptom-free existence on a higher dose that promises a shorter efficacy period.

As Irene's narrative in the chapter introduction shows, sufferers early in their experience of the disorder are often relieved and satisfied by the medications. This early disposition is known as the "medication honeymoon"—a period when the dismay at diagnosis is alleviated by the promise of symptomatic relief. But after a decade of carbidopa-levodopa, the wearing-off syndrome may present. Wearing off refers to the loss of function between doses. PD sufferers become beholden to this medication window—the time between doses when their abilities are restored. In the early stage, sufferers may be taking carbidopa-levodopa twice daily, but as their disorder progresses they may find themselves medicating as often as every two hours. As Leroy's episode in the hardware store illustrates (chapter 1), sufferers with moderate or severe PD must plan and schedule activities around their "on" times, or they may face embarrassing consequences. This does not mean that reliance upon levodopa necessitates a relinquishment of control. Support group discussions frequently emphasized the importance of negotiating the dosages and timing of levodopa pills with a neurologist. This negotiation maximizes and matches the "on" periods with activities or times that are meaningful for each person. The challenges of medication management lie not only in restoring motor function, but also in maintaining a balance between function and side effects, notably freezing and dyskinesia.

The medication window gradually shortens over time but is relatively predictable. Freezing, a transitory lack of motor function control, is not predictable. While most often implicated in gait problems, freezing can occur in other motor functions as well. PD sufferers have developed a wide range of cues to "unfreeze" themselves. They count off steps as if marching, they take a step backward, they run a few steps, or they place strips of tape across the floor to visually break up the space that they are navigating. Some walkers now come equipped with small laser pointers that the user can shine on the floor to facilitate smoother walking. Freezing is the source of much unpredictability in the embodiment of PD. As Hazel, a married woman in her eighties, summarized, "So I don't know what I'm running into, you know. And the thing is, you never know. The thing you can't do one day, you can the next. Or in less time than that. And that's—that's a little disturbing in that you're never sure what you can do." Freezing becomes yet another condition affecting sufferers' experience, but one they cannot control.

Many sufferers consider carbidopa-levodopa the source of dyskinesias, or involuntary movements, and dystonias, stiff and sometimes painful twisting of the limbs, hands, or feet (Vernon 1989). Dyskinesias are unsettling to witness and can be painful, embarrassing, or even dangerous. I had first seen dyskinesia in action while watching the actor and PD activist Michael J. Fox discuss stem cell research on television. His arms, shoulders, and head moved in an uncoordinated, disconcerting fashion. Despite having seen this phenomenon before, my initial responses to witnessing dyskinesia in the field were surprise and alarm. I watched PD patients stagger, walk into walls, fall out of chairs, spill beverages, struggle with their coat sleeves, and hold conversations despite bobbing heads and spasming shoulders. I learned to be preemptive with doors and chairs and how and when to offer my assistance. Levodopa users share a common dread of dyskinesia, because it is uncontrollable and frequently unpredictable, makes them appear to be drunk or mentally ill, and significantly, signals the limitations of current pharmacotherapy. Freezing and dyskinesia frame PD as a condition of loss of control, either in stillness or movement.

Because of the medication window and dyskinesia, some PD sufferers considered the decision to start carbidopa-levodopa a life-changing event. As Jeanne explains, having to take medications to restore function made her feel older than her sixty-seven years and more dependent than she was ready to experience:

> I just want to be independent, and at first I wasn't even taking my meds when [the doctor] gave them to me. He prescribed carbidopa-levodopa three times a day. I would take one in the morning (I never took drugs), and I would forget the noon one and then I would take the evening one. So then I came in to see him and he said that he was going to increase my dosage. And I said, "Doctor, I'm not even taking the three; don't increase it!" And he was very angry at me.

Bonnie, sixty-three and ten years postdiagnosis, continues to work full-time and aimed to wait at least ten years before taking this medication.

SAMANTHA: Did [your doctor] start you on carbidopa-levodopa right away?

BONNIE: No. I have just had it about two years now. I did selegiline at first. I did that for quite a while—about five years, I would say. And then we added a lower dose of pramipexole dihydrochloride. . . . Then [my doctor] suggested that I add the carbidopa-levodopa. And I said, "I don't want to do that. I don't want to take it yet." And he said, "Well, whenever you are ready, here is the scrip for it."

SAMANTHA: Why didn't you want to take it?

BONNIE: [My doctor] asked me that, too. I said, "Well, I guess I feel like that's the end of the end." That's the last medication. I kept having other medications that I could add and improve my situation. When I get to carbidopa-levodopa, there are no more to improve it. So then what's going to happen? How long before . . . ? Well, I finally got over that and decided that I didn't like the quality of life I had. It was really deteriorating. I was really slow. It wasn't a very normal feeling I had. . . . I just wanted a better quality of life than what I was having. I went ahead and went on it. . . . I said that I had always wanted to at least make ten years before I would try it. That was my magic number before I started [carbidopa-levodopa]. I was hoping that I could, but I didn't.

Bonnie had experienced increasing bouts of balance problems, falling, freezing events, and tremor leading up to her decision to initiate therapy. On the medication her symptoms were much improved, but she decided to make the trade-off between regaining better function and possibly reaching the end of the pharmaceutical armamentarium in favor of quality of life.

Medication Management: Somatic and Social Implications of Adding to the Mix

Levodopa has its strengths and limitations but remains the primary medication to treat PD symptoms among older PD sufferers. Anticholinergics, dopamine receptor agonists, amantadine, monoamine oxidase inhibitors (MAO-B inhibitors), and catechol-o-methyltransferase inhibitors (COMT inhibitors) are frequently prescribed in concert with levodopa preparations or as a stand-alone treatment to forestall levodopa use. Each of these classes of medications presents different costs and benefits.

Anticholinergics target rigidity and bradykinesia and are used in addition to levodopa to further address motor symptoms (Chung, Wu, and Lew 2003). They are associated with hallucinations and confusion, so their use among elders is limited. Dopamine agonists have been used to treat PD since the 1970s, but the two most common DAs, pramipexole and ropinerole, were only recently approved for use in the United States (Stacy 2003). Unlike levodopa, which must be converted to dopamine by the body, DAs act directly upon dopamine receptors in the brain. DAs are often prescribed as a stand-alone therapy for younger onset PD patients, as in Bonnie's case, prolonging the amount of time before they begin levodopa use. Among elders, DAs are more commonly prescribed in concert with levodopa; this approach reduces the consumption of both medications. Amantadine is an antiviral agent that works by increasing the release of dopamine in the brain and may be neuroprotective (Chung, Wu, and Lew 2003). Its efficacy in treating PD symptoms is somewhat modest, and its potential to cause urinary retention and confusion make it contraindicated for older men. MAO-B inhibitors help the body by making dopamine more available for uptake. They can be used as a monotherapy in early PD, but are more commonly used as an adjunct treatment with levodopa in later stages (Victor and Waters 2003). MAO-B inhibitors can decrease the amount of levodopa necessary to achieve symptomatic relief, but their use is contraindicated for persons who are taking certain antidepressants. They may also increase dyskinesia. COMT inhibitors are taken with levodopa to increase its longevity in the body. They may decrease the overall use of levodopa and help patients who experience end-of-dose problems (Pfeiffer 2003). All these medications, whether used as first-line or adjunct therapies, produce side effects, many of which worsen in severity with age. These side effects include hallucinations, unexpected sleeping episodes, and compulsive gambling. Such side effects have considerable negative influence upon a user's quality of life.

Hallucinations, while not commonly reported by PD sufferers, were often brought up by caregivers at support group meetings and during interviews.

PD medications are not solely to blame for hallucinations but are well-known sources of them. June, a divorced woman in her eighties with moderate PD, has dealt with hallucinations of varying severity for a few years. Despite her ability, in retrospect, to recognize them as such, these "waking dreams," as I learned to finesse them, can pose serious consequences. Most commonly PD medications cause sufferers to hallucinate small animals and children, but even these seemingly positive visions are quite disturbing to both sufferers and their partners, as June explains.

> [My doctor] tried several different [medications]. They didn't work. One of them gave me hallucinations. It was really weird, because there were three times that I'd hear a loud knock on my door. It was usually between two and four in the morning. I have a peephole in my door. I got up and looked out to see if I could see anybody. There were usually two people there. And I gave the police a good description. [laughs] I called the sheriff. Last time, [the man I saw] had a knife and he was saying, "You know what I am going to do with this when I get in there? I am going to kill you!" That was scary. I called the sheriff and they checked the apartment building out, and I knew which apartments were empty, and they went in there and checked but never could find anybody. I felt like calling the sheriff and apologizing, but I didn't have the nerve. [laughs]

Hallucinations were a source of disagreements between Richard and Lorraine, a married couple who have lived together in their small bungalow for more than forty years. Richard had been forced to retire earlier than he had wanted to because of executive function and memory problems. Lorraine handles all his medications. In this context, she raised the topic of hallucinations.

LORRAINE: Right now he's not on as many [medications]. He's on donepezil HCL and quetiapine fumarate at bedtime and then he's on venlaflaxine HCL and the regular carbidopa-levodopa [two pills three times per day]. Those are the only PD ones that he's on right now. The entacapone he came off of, because he was having hallucinations and stuff.

He was having [hallucinations] almost throughout the whole day and night. Most of it was seeing people. People were always in the house. Well, he still has them occasionally, but not near what that was. That was just a little too much. I guess I was the one that couldn't handle it. [To Richard] Because it didn't bother you.

RICHARD: I think you are right.

LORRAINE: It was, you know, "There's people in the house all of the time." One time he did get pretty belligerent. That's when I really got concerned. You had claimed that there were people down in the basement and that they wouldn't leave; that was it. And he was just so riled up that night. He was going to call the cops. Have the cops come out.

RICHARD: They were here, too.

LORRAINE: No, they weren't.

RICHARD: Not the cops, no.

LORRAINE: No, but there wasn't anybody here, either.

RICHARD: They came in the . . . when the first people came, they sat down there and the women crocheted.

LORRAINE: See, he comes up with all of these things, and he doesn't believe me when I keep saying that there's nobody here. Sometimes I have to say, "Yeah, fine. Whatever." [laughs] Because he still has some.

Similar to Gordon and Irene early in this chapter, Richard and Lorraine differ as to the frequency and veracity of hallucinations. This becomes a frequent basis for arguments between spouses, leading caregivers to sleep with one eye open and PD sufferers to feel infantilized by their spouse's negation of their visions. Hallucinations were perhaps more problematic for PD patients who lived alone and had no one to rein them in when their version of reality might endanger them. As June told me, she didn't "have the nerve" to call the sheriff and apologize because she knew that her confession would lead to an intensification of the pressure she already received from her family to move into a nursing home. June was able to laugh about the incident now that months had passed, but her vision was very frightening and the consequences of being "caught" very real.

Antipsychotics and antidepressants are commonly used in more advanced or in akinetic PD cases to alleviate the frequency and strain of hallucinations. It is difficult for elders to admit to cognitive or mental health problems, and challenging for health care providers to find ways to treat cognitive sequelae associated with PD. Depression, dementia, anxiety, psychosis, confusion, delusions, and agitation can all occur with PD. PD, aging, comorbidities, and medication use can all contribute to nonmotor problems of PD patients. Separating out the ultimate cause of these symptoms from the possible sources is a complex diagnostic maze. Physicians must first rule out a coexisting urinary tract or other infection (Starkstein and Merello 2002). Once that has been ruled out, the balancing act of titrating enough PD medication to restore function while administering as conservative a dose as possible begins. Decreasing PD medications may increase dyskinesia and rigidity, while increasing them may cause psychosis. Patient age, longevity of disease, gender, genetics, and a host of other variables all conspire to create a unique response to medications. The addition of a particular DA may cause psychosis that remits when it is removed. Alternately, physicians may elect to add another medication to treat cognitive symptoms. However, many elders refused to take medications billed as "antide-pressants" or "antipsychotics." As Ella, a sixty-year-old caregiver told me:

> My husband doesn't like the quetiapine fumarate recently prescribed since he learned it is an antipsychotic. I have a difficult time getting him to take it. He's very clear that it isn't because of side effects, but because of the general use for this type of medicine. He's also angry with his doctor for prescribing it and considers finding a new doctor. I'm curious whether this is just my husband, or if it occurs with others as their disease advances or begins to cause mental confusion. If I could direct research I'd seek solutions to the advanced symptoms, selfishly, because I don't know how to help my husband as his condition worsens.

When these same medications were simply framed as "PD drugs," they were more willingly accepted.

Treating cognitive symptoms is also difficult because elders may tolerate antidepressants or antipsychotics poorly (Schrag 2004). But the successful treatment of cognitive symptoms (or side effects) depends upon a physician's knowledge of their occurrence. Some people strive to schedule their appointments during their best "on" periods. Unless a health care provider directly inquires about such symptoms or a caregiver reports them, physicians may not be cognizant of their patients' psychotic episodes. Hallucination sufferers downplayed their power and frequency, but their caregivers became animated, contesting their partner's report. Interestingly, some PD patients never divulged to me that they experienced cognitive problems, but they reported the use of antipsychotic medications on their questionnaires.

Conversation about medications invariably included a tour of the household medication shoebox. Interviewees would drag out their shoebox of pill bottles (sometimes with bravado) and show me firsthand which ones they took and how many of each. If someone pulled out something like amitriptyline, I would ask what it was for. Rather than reference sleeping or depression, most people would simply say that it was for their PD. Of course, they were right, but the lack of disclosure, intentional or not, illustrated to me both the stigma of mental health conditions and the skill of physicians who navigated around the stigma to find a socially acceptable way to entice their patients to comply with treatment.

Unexpected sleeping episodes and compulsive gambling were far less frequently reported than hallucinations, but these also demonstrate the ways in which medications can become another set of conditions upon sufferers' lives. "Unexpected sleep episodes" are a kind of narcolepsy associated with the use of DAs (Stacy 2003). These episodes commonly occur during daytime hours when sufferers are trying to enjoy a social event. They unexpectedly and uncontrollably fall asleep, missing much of the wedding, baseball game, or meeting they were attending and waking up to an offended party and embarrassment. Sufferers reported feeling that others viewed their sleeping as a sign of cognitive incompetence, and they fought the narcolepsy both to participate in desirable events and to forestall suspicions of dementia. I witnessed numerous instances of these sleeping events and had to learn not to take it personally when someone dropped off in the midst of a conversation. While I at times had to make sure that the sleeper wasn't going to fall out of their chair, I wondered how they fared when on their own, without the watchful eye of an interested party. Bonnie, whose decision to begin levodopa therapy was discussed earlier, suffered from a serious car accident due to an unexpected sleep episode. She dropped off to sleep while she was driving on a rural highway and awoke heading toward a car in the oncoming lane. Bonnie overcorrected and her car landed upside down in a ditch. She escaped this incident with minor injuries, but she was not permitted to drive again until she was able to get her medications under control.

Compulsive gambling is perhaps the most unusual medication side effect that PD sufferers must contend with. At the time of my fieldwork, the medical community was just beginning to understand the connection between medications and this socially aberrant behavior. Until that time it was thought that there was something unique about PD sufferers' personality that compelled them to gamble recklessly. Anyone who has lived in Iowa for any length of time would certainly find this laughable. Of course, there are persons for whom gambling can be an addictive and pathological behavior, but on the whole this sort of activity does not sit well with the heartland Christian ethos. Pramipexole and ropinerole, both DAs, have been implicated in compulsive gambling (Singh et al. 2007); these cases are more common among men. DAs are also thought to activate other latent compulsive behaviors such as overeating or hypersexuality. I met two female caregivers who confided in me that their husbands had secretly gambled away their life savings, forcing them to sell possessions to pay bills. And one support group meeting focused on one man's efforts to spread the word among PD sufferers that his experience with gambling could happen to them—that such behavior was not a sign of moral weakness but a biochemical chain reaction.

From Ablation to Stimulation: Surgical Approaches

Surgical approaches are treatments of last resort for PD—they are expensive, invasive, and limited to the most severely affected sufferers under the age of seventy. Neurosurgical treatment of PD has been around since the 1960s, but recent research has dramatically changed its underlying theory, complexity, and outcomes. Early surgical interventions, namely pallidotomy and thalamotomy, used ablative techniques to apply lesions on the brain in the affected areas. Pallidotomy applies lesions to the globus pallidum and is indicated for the reduction of levodopa-induced dyskinesias and dystonias (Fischer 1999; Lang and Lozano 1998b). Thalamotomy is thought to relieve tremor and rigidity by targeting the thalamus (Duvoisin and Sage 1996). The benefits of ablative techniques depend upon the location of the lesion and the severity of symptoms involved. Though the efficacy of ablative surgeries has improved since their inception, they are no longer the most popular neurosurgical intervention. Ablative techniques can worsen existing symptoms or create new limitations. Unlike medications and newer surgical interventions, ablation surgeries create permanent neuroanatomical changes (Samuel and Lang 2003).

About one-third of the way through my fieldwork, several support group meetings turned their focus to a surgical treatment for PD recently approved by the Federal Drug Administration—deep brain stimulation (DBS). What had been an experimental therapy at the beginning of my research on PD now possesses FDA approval and is eligible for Medicare and VHA reimbursement. It is now the most common form of surgical intervention for PD (Samuel and Lang 2003). DBS differs from ablative techniques in its precision and reversibility. In DBS, one or two electrodes are implanted into the brain to supply ongoing "chronic electrical stimulation" to relieve motor-related symptoms (Kirschstein 2000). The electrodes are connected by wires that run under the scalp and down the neck to a battery and programming unit located just below the breastbone. The neurologist can program these units remotely using an electrical device. DBS's therapeutic efficacy depends upon the electrodes' location, frequency, and intensity, as well as on patient characteristics such as their age or the severity of their symptoms. In light of the cultural and medical gravity associated with neurosurgery, DBS is not lightly undertaken. Patients with moderate cognitive impairment or dementia or who are over the age of seventy are generally ineligible for the procedure. DBS candidates risk infection (at the stimulator lead or cranial wound sites), the potential that their symptoms will worsen after surgery, and death. Patients must undergo general anesthesia during the stimulator implantation and battery replacement, which presents health risks. DBS has been associated with intracranial hemorrhage, infection of the stimulator leads, lead migration, and organic rejection of the hardware (Pahwa and Lyons 2003).

With this information in mind, I was slightly disturbed by the sales pitches of the pharmaceutical representatives who frequented PD support groups. They screened short films with dramatic before-and-after images that made DBS seem a panacea for PD. I rarely heard them discuss the high cost of DBS, though they did mention that Medicare would cover it. Nor did they broadcast the age limit for surgery—most of the support group attendees would be considered too old for DBS.

Nine people who participated in my study reported having had neurosurgery, and eight of these had undergone DBS implantation. My conversations with DBS patients reveal both its magic and its limitations. For these sufferers, DBS was a last chance for relief from the side effects of intense polypharmacy. All eight DBS patients had PD in their forties and underwent surgery in their fifties or sixties. Postsurgery, all still had prominent PD symptoms and relied upon numerous PD medications. Nonetheless, DBS was a transformative experience. Patients are awake during the sometimes ten-hour-long surgery, their heads immobilized by a large steel frame screwed into their scalp (under a local anesthetic). Small, nickel-sized holes are drilled into the skull to access the brain, and the micro-thin electrical leads are placed in the brain. Patients are asked to respond to questions during this process in order to verify the correct position of the electrodes. The stimulators are turned on anywhere from six weeks to three months after the surgery, to allow time for recovery. Patients are given remote controls that they can use to turn the system off or on. They are also warned that strong magnetic fields can disrupt DBS performance; sometimes simply opening the refrigerator shuts the system off.

Eileen decided to have DBS surgery when her dyskinesia was so severe that she could barely maintain her balance to sit in a chair. I interviewed her two years after her surgery, and she continues to live with some severe mobility impairments. While Eileen's dyskinesia had improved so much that she is now able to play the piano again, her ambulatory competence has decreased. I posed this change to her as a trade-off; she had gained in her ability to control her movement, but she had lost a great deal of her balance and ability to walk. Eileen disagreed with my characterization. Instead of viewing the postsurgical deterioration of her walking as a side effect, she interpreted it as disease progression. She asserted that she would undergo DBS surgery again, despite her disturbing descriptions of the surgical process and her deteriorating physical health. Eileen must now use a wheelchair to traverse any distance and in general cannot walk unassisted. In my original estimation I had assumed that this was a meaningful loss to her sense of self-control and identity. However, Eileen's regained ability to prepare basic meals, write, and play the piano were significant to her sense of well-being and self expression. In this case, I found myself learning to recognize my own biases concerning the impact and meaning of disability and was reminded to define such somatic experiences in an autobiographical, life course perspective.

Wallace's experience after surgery differed from Eileen's. He also had severe dyskinesia and was on high doses of carbidopa-levodopa. He used a motorized wheelchair to get around town and could no longer drive. I met Wallace at the start of my fieldwork, when he had just begun to pursue DBS surgery. He went through months of neuropsychiatric testing and evaluation before he was approved for the procedure. His DBS was an event in the local PD community. Other group members confided in me that they felt bad for Wallace and hoped that they wouldn't end up like him, but they were excited for his impending recovery with DBS. But Wallace's experience did not live up to the glossy results that the pharmaceutical company representative's films celebrated. His symptoms did improve somewhat. Wallace was able to walk almost a block without his wheelchair, and his speech intelligibility improved slightly. But he still had to take massive doses of carbidopa-levodopa. He was disappointed by the modest improvements DBS provided, and he was floored when one of his surgical sites became infected. Wallace had to undergo surgery a second time and have the leads removed. After more than a year of testing and advocating for the surgery, he was in worse shape than when he started.

Eileen's and Wallace's cases represent the limitations of DBS. The other DBS patients in this study had better experiences. Their symptoms improved dramatically, as the promotional films promised, and their medication use decreased. Better able to tolerate levodopa, and struggling with less dyskinesia, they were living examples of DBS's magic. Fellow support group members would remark to me on the improvement that DBS had wrought. Everyone who had undergone DBS still looked to me like they had PD, with their slowed movement and stiff expressions, but their suffering was greatly decreased. These success stories were the topic of many proud and excited discussions among fellow support group members, but the experiences of those for whom DBS was ineffective were little discussed, and these people were at times objects of pity.

Complementary and Alternative Modalities for PD Relief

The literature on complementary and alternative medicine (CAM) treatment of PD spans several modalities. One of the earliest descriptions of PD appears in Ayurvedic texts, which have thirty-five treatments for the disease (Manyam and Sanchez-Ramos 1999). Select herbal remedies used in Chinese medicine have been associated with symptomatic improvement in clinical settings (Manyam and Sanchez-Ramos 1999). Rajendran, Thompson, and Reich (2001) found that 40 percent of PD patients recruited from a university-based movement disorders clinic reported using at least one CAM for PD symptoms. Significantly, a recent study of older adults enrolled in a Medicare program notes that patients neither disclose their CAM usage to physicians nor do they gain information about such CAMs from scientific sources (Astin et al. 2000).

Overall, there has been little scientific study of the efficacy of CAM therapies in PD treatment, and scant attention to whether and to what extent PD sufferers might utilize them (Chrischilles et al. 1998; Manyam and Sanchez-Ramos 1999). A population-based study conducted in Iowa found that 45 percent of PD sufferers used ancillary services; of these, 20 percent used chiropractors and 18 percent visited physical therapists (Chrischilles et al. 1998). Similarly, questionnaire respondents in my study reported limited use of allied health providers. The low incidence of CAM use by PD patients in this study may be due to several factors: (1) a reluctance to divulge such use for fear of being judged or fear that their behavior would offend either me or their physician; (2) limited economic resources to pay for CAM treatment; and (3) limited knowledge of the available CAM modalities or disbelief in their efficacy. Physicians are more likely to prescribe levodopa than massage or physical therapy, and I once heard a neurologist refer to the most commonly used CAM, over-the-counter vitamins, as a "waste of time."

Although I did not collect any data specifically pertaining to religious practice, faith is an integral coping mechanism of the Iowan PD sufferers with whom I worked. My involvement in support groups and individual families' lives brought me closer to their faith communities and belief systems than I had expected. Reflective of the entire state of Iowa, only a handful of Jewish families participated in the study. A majority of participants were Catholics or Protestants. Of all the treatments available, prayer and faith were the least expensive, with no known side effects or risks. More than half of sufferers reported prayer as a treatment for symptoms.

Chiropractic and massage were the next most commonly cited modalities, but on further investigation, these were used not routinely but for short-term treatment of acute back pain. Next to prayer, the most widely used CAM was over-the-counter vitamins. Vitamins were viewed as innocuous dietary supplements that could only improve health. About 30 percent of PD sufferers used a supplement without the express recommendation of a doctor. Vitamin E, considered by some to be neuroprotective in PD, was the most widely used supplement. Only a few people used the more recently touted Coenzyme Q10 (CoQ10) supplement; most people had never even heard of it. One person used a natural form of levodopa purchased through the mail. When asked if supplements helped with particular PD symptoms, everyone told me that they are supposed to help by slowing progression. Only one person told me that they could see a difference in their own body.

How Do You Treat a Condition?

Medication management is a major thread in the PD research literature. How can we get PD sufferers to improve their self-care? To adhere to medications? What is the best pharmacotherapy for particular symptoms, ages, or stages of PD? Such questions spring from positive concern for the well-being of PD sufferers, but they reflect a disconnect from the lived experience of PD as a condition. Management of this multisystem disorder is complex, and sufferers seem to go through stages of adjusting to it. As Irene's sardonic narrative shows, early in the disorder sufferers may view the large PD pharmacopoeia as positive. Their grief at being diagnosed with a terrible disorder is attenuated by the existence of so many medications to treat it. This relief is subsequently tempered by the lack of a clear association between the disorder and a single medication. Many sufferers expect that they will be offered one medication to treat their one disorder. What they find is that they are offered one medication to treat their primary condition or symptom, and that as new conditions arise they are offered additional medicines. As their personal regimen increases in complexity, they are further offered new medications to address the side effects of earlier ones. Thus, it is unsurprising that many sufferers take more than one dozen different medications daily—and a sizable number take close to twenty different medications daily to treat both PD and comorbid disorders.

The process of arriving at a medication regimen is one of experimentation in the most positive sense: Physicians must be attuned to the individual needs of their patient in order to mutually discover the best treatment at a given time. But this process rarely enhances sufferers' feelings of being well taken care of; rather, many of them describe feeling that there should be a simpler, more exacting method for treating PD. They could not understand why, in a room of ten PD sufferers, each will be on different medications, dosages, and regimens. That being said, the experimentation process of determining the best match of medicines to conditions is viewed differently depending on who is directing it. When PD sufferers take titrating into their own hands, they often do so in secret and in resistance to their physician's advice. In these instances they assert a sense of agency over their own lives, in resistance to the fatalism that accompanies the prospect of a lifelong dependence on medicines.

Medication use is nonnegotiable and heightens participants' sense of disorder. Their medications do not always work, the dosages are frequently readjusted, they have numerous side effects, and their longevity of use is limited. Sufferers' dependence upon medication is compounded by their need for assistance from their spouses in managing them. Compliance issues with levodopa exacerbate this. For maximum efficacy, carbidopa-levodopa doses should be taken within an hour of their prescribed time. For some patients this is every two hours; for others it is every eight hours. The frequency may serve as a constant reminder of dependence. Medications have to be set aside in compartmentalized boxes, organized by day of the week and time of the day. They must be picked up at the store and paid for. Insurance forms must be filed. And most importantly, patients need to remember to take them. Treatment demands represent yet another way in which PD functions as a condition on elders' embodiment of aging. In the later stages of PD, sufferers' lives can come to be organized around treatments, rather than their treatments orchestrated around their individual desires.

Treatments set a condition on sufferers' future plans as well. Sufferers must consider not only the long-term effects of individual drugs, but also the economic consequences of increasing out-of-pocket medication expenses. The recent Medicare Part D plan had only recently been implemented when I was in the field. Despite advertising to the contrary, very few elders had confidence that the plan would lessen the economic hardship of PD drugs. Many suspected that it would actually worsen their situation by allowing their private prescription plans to drop or reduce existing coverage because of the availability of government-sponsored assistance. For elders living on a fixed income, medication expenses were sizable and worrisome. For younger sufferers still in the workforce, the need for prescription coverage and insurance added to their concerns that they might be forced out of work before they were eligible for Medicare.

Therapeutic management of PD, then, is another lens through which we can understand the space between sickness and health in the case of PD. Medications themselves can be seen as a stand-in for the condition, a frequent physical reminder that one is not an independent autonomous agent or someone who just feels "sick." Sufferers are initially entranced by the medication honeymoon and then brought to understand the medication window as a new condition upon their lives. As such, medications underscore the ways in which PD demands attention, is unpredictable, and portends an ambiguous future.

7

It Gets Worse

Introduction: Planning for the Unpredictable

Anna was born and raised on a farm just outside a small town in southern Iowa. She met her husband to be, Thomas, at a country dance when they were teenagers, and they married just a few years later. Anna stayed at home with her children until the youngest was in school. At that time she began a career in clerical and accounting positions at various companies in more urban areas of the state. Anna and her husband retired the same week about twenty years ago and have been enjoying this phase of married life, although recent years have unfolded differently than they had imagined.

About ten years ago Thomas noticed that Anna's facial demeanor was changing: She was beginning to resemble her father, who suffered with severe PD in the years before medications were available. They sought the opinion of a university neurologist, who confirmed their suspicions. Anna remarked on this troubling news. "I think I handled it pretty good, even after they told me that I had it. I just did the best I could. They said, 'If you get depressed [there are treatments]' but I didn't. Like now, I mean, as things are getting to be where [there's] less that I can do. I can't drive and more things that I can't do, it adds up to the depression side."

Anna's symptoms are primarily akinetic. At seventy-four, she is slow, fatigues easily, sleeps often, has balance impairments which affect her walking, and finds herself confused by once unremarkable, familiar tasks. She increasingly relies upon Thomas's help, which causes her distress at the same time that she expresses gratitude for his continuing affection. "Oh, there's a lot of stuff he don't let me do that I think I could do," she says. "He's so afraid that I could get burned [by the stove] or hurt. He has taken over cooking. . . . But he takes good care of me."

For Thomas's part, the PD has introduced him to new household responsibilities and pressures. He told me, "Anna's easy to work with. The thing is, she always tries to do her share yet, but you know [she can't]. I let her do what she can, sometimes. . . . I think two years ago I started noticing when we were driving, I would see things and say, 'Did you see that?' and she'd say no, and they would be right next to her. As things progressed I said to her, 'I really don't feel comfortable letting you drive anymore. I am afraid that you are going to get hurt or hurt somebody.' And she agreed. I'll tell you what I did. She felt so bad and she cried about giving up [driving] and I understand that. I took her out to the ballpark out here where there's a big open area to drive. I set her behind the wheel and she couldn't even get the car moving." These days Thomas does all the yard work, housework, meals, finances, and socializing.

This is not the life Anna and Thomas expected to have in retirement. The first ten years, prior to the PD diagnosis, they spent traveling, fishing, dining out with friends, reading, and working on crafts and other hobbies. Now, Anna says:

> I don't feel like I can do too much of anything, really. For a while I was doing the washing and folding the clothes. I can do that. I can dust the floor. This thing is, I don't have enough strength to keep going. Say I get a couple of things done, like vacuuming or something, and I am all done, aren't I? Just like now, I am getting real tired. I have to lay my head down and go to sleep. [laughs] It's limited me in just about anything. [All I do is] eat and sleep. . . . And I am not good at doing crafts or doing anything. I used to be able to crochet. I got like this and I tried to crochet, but I can't even do it.

Thomas tries to encourage her and tells me, "She's been getting up in the morning and making breakfast." Anna discounts his effort, embarrassed. "Making Instant Breakfast, boy, that's a hard thing to do." She laughs. "Sometimes I get mixed up. Like making oatmeal, it's like I forgot how to do it." Thomas reaches over and puts his hand on her arm. "It's all right," he says.

He turns to me with a glance that acknowledges our shared understanding of Anna's limitations and of his awkward attempts to spare her feelings. Thomas tells me:

> Well, our life has changed a lot. I am saying this in a positive way, because we were retired for ten years. We did a lot of traveling with the RV and we had a lot of fun. And then when I started to see these symptoms, why we went down there and had it diagnosed. She started taking medication right away. I think that's helped her to get an early start on it. . . . We are getting in a position now where I am starting to look for someplace to move to. I've had bypass surgery and I am not strong enough to lift her if I need to and stuff. And I see things happening. I'd rather look ahead than be forced to make a quick decision. I have gotten together with our attorney and we are getting things set up so that she can enter into the decisions we are making together, so that I don't have to make all of them.

I have that set up for later on. I've talked to them a couple of times. I want to do the best job I can in taking care of things that way, as long as she knows what's going on.

I don't want to do anything that upsets her. You drove by the adult day care [on your way here]. I didn't like to leave her [alone at home] because I didn't want her . . . she might have the stove on and put her hand on it or something. I ask her not to run anything when I am gone— dishwasher, mixer, or anything like that. She can run the microwave; I don't think that can hurt her. So I took her down [to the adult day care] one day. She wanted me to stay. Finally after a couple of hours [a staff person asked him to leave]. And I did and I got home and I was in trouble. Because she was so upset. She said that I took her down there and abandoned her. And she cried and cried and cried. I said, you know, we'll just have to wait on that part of it.

It took months of encouragement from family to get Thomas to explore the possibility of adult day care. Anna's response to her first day broke his heart, and he waited another six months before attempting it again. Thomas struggles to maintain the integrity of their partnership, approaching Anna as an equal even as her abilities falter. They want to maintain their current residence for as long as possible, and it is hard to imagine Thomas reconciling himself to long-term care. He rarely leaves the house without Anna because he is afraid that she will try to use the stove or fall, but taking her to the grocery store makes a thirty-minute errand into one that could take more than two hours. At the core, Thomas and Anna's plan for retirement has not changed: They are spending more and more time together enjoying the solitude of their home and each other's company. However, the shift in the balance of responsibilities and the increased social isolation have taken their toll, too. Anna resists it for herself, but Thomas is now seeing a counselor for support.

When considering relocating to a smaller home with less upkeep or even an assisted-living apartment, Thomas must also weigh whether and for how long they could afford such a change. Financial decisions have emerged as a particularly tough issue, as their medication expenses topped $7,000 the previous year. One of Anna's medications can cost more than $150 per day. For the time being, they are able to acquire it from a Canadian pharmacy, through technically illegal but unregulated means. When the loophole closes, Anna will have to find another PD treatment that relieves her symptoms but does not aggravate her stomach. Thomas and Anna are able to pay for their increasing medical bills by drawing on two small IRAs and their savings account, but the viability of this plan depends upon Anna's PD progressing at a slow rate, with few new medications and no need of outside services. For now, retired life for Anna is a drama of competing emotional scripts, ranging from resentful to grateful to resigned to depressed. Her plans for travel and her social life have dissipated. For Thomas, retirement is as busy as working life once was, yet for different reasons than he expected. Now, instead of waking early to fish, he wakes early to get a start on the day's housework, and his calendar is crowded with doctor's appointments rather than dates with friends.

Progression and Prognosis

PD is considered to be a progressive condition, but the rate of progression differs from person to person. Progression from mild to severe PD may occur over the course of several years or even decades. Symptomatology and disease presentation have been used to predict progression, but recent studies imply that age at onset is a greater factor (Alves et al. 2005). The older one is at onset, the more rapidly the disease progresses (Alves et al. 2005; Meara and Bhowmick 2000). So, in the words of one man, what do older PD sufferers have "to look forward to"?

There have been many efforts to create disease-stage models for PD. The first and most widely used (and modified) is the five-stage scale devised by Hoehn and Yahr (1967). At the first stage, unilateral disease, persons have symptoms that affect one side of the body. Stage two, bilateral disease, marks the progression of PD symptoms to both sides of the body. Stage three adds postural instability—PD sufferers who are experiencing accidental falls and moderate impairment from akinesia or tremor. Stage four describes very impaired persons with severe gait and balance disabilities. Persons in stage five are often wheelchair bound or bedridden and may also have had a tracheotomy, gastrostomy, or both to address swallowing impairments.

These stages are useful for understanding the range of potentialities and for conducting clinical studies, but the heterogeneity of PD means that each person experiences the disease uniquely. The appearance of symptoms does not always follow this neat order. For example, swallowing difficulties may occur prior to gait impairments, or visual disturbances may predate hallucinations or dementia.

Newly diagnosed PD sufferers often respond to explanations of these stages with trepidation and anxiety. Rather than view progression scales as a range of possible outcomes, many sufferers and caregivers see them as a road map for the future. People come to accept progression as their definitive prognosis and believe that they will never improve and will inevitably decline. This is not the case with Helen. "They say its slow progressing. I think Harry, maybe, was saying, 'It damned well doesn't seem very slow to me!' I have determined, of course, that it is quite slow. It's just that by the time we know it, then it seems like it is going really fast. . . . If you could actually say that it started when I was thirty-five, say, I am sixty-three today. Well, I am just pretty darned good, aren't I? It's just that saying seven years [ago] that I could put all this stuff on the shelves and now I can't get on a ladder. That seems like real rapid progression then."

More typical was this dialogue with an eighy-one-year-old:

SAMANTHA: Do you feel like your Parkinson's is getting worse?

RALPH: Yes. It is slow. I have nothing to look forward to. The bad part is coming, but it is slow.

A comment in a similar vein came from a PD sufferer who laughed when he told me, "I am seventy-six so I am hoping that by the time it starts getting bad that I will kick the bucket."

This sense of the disease's inevitable downward progression, despite its unpredictable course, pervaded all contexts of the research. Support group meetings were monthly markers, and members would assess their colleagues' function with a keen eye toward progression. Remarks such as, "You see people who are worse off than you are and it helps you to be thankful," or "I find groups depressing because they remind me of what is in store for me," were commonly shared with me in private conversation (see chapter 8). One caregiver said to me, "When we told one of my cousins that [my husband] had PD, his immediate response was, 'What a cruel disease.' And it is, as it progresses. But, you know, we just have learned to take one day at a time. We try to make the best of each day that we have. . . . And we can always look around and see somebody who is worse off than we are. So we are always thankful for what we have."

Like the support group members, I marked progression in individual people from month to month, and in a few cases until they no longer attended meetings because they were too disabled or because they had died. Being a witness to participants' physical decline is a heavy emotional responsibility that became more profound as the months passed. Each support group had at least one member who I feared would die before the year was out, but rarely were my feelings correct. Underscoring the irrationality of this remarkable disorder is the unpredictability of decline. Sometimes men and women who seemed the most vigorous, engaged, happy, and well functioning of the group experienced substantial decline in just one month's time. Besides the usual age-associated suspects—stroke, COPD, and heart failure—people's bodies succumbed to the sequelae of PD symptoms: pneumonia from aspirating food or death from a fall or car accident. PD sufferers laugh darkly at the books that assert: "No one dies from PD," for they recognize that PD symptoms contribute to premature death.

Interviews with people about their feelings on their prognosis and disease course reveal a wealth of emotions. Common to many sicknesses, a sufferer's stance on progression can reflect humor, ambivalence, denial, fear, anger, and acceptance. Only a very few people had expected to develop PD, and so a majority had made retirement plans based on their health at the time. One plans for retirement knowing that old age will arrive one day, but few people plan to spend their retirement filling prescriptions and wondering how long they have until they become physically dependent upon others. However mild the case, all

PD sufferers must address these concerns and make sense of them in the context of their current age, functional status, and social life.

Recognizing Progression and Prognosis

Progression is ascribed meaning based on such demographic variables as sufferer's age, socioeconomic status, and marital status, but it also derives meaning from the values attributed to particular activities and the extent to which people are no longer able to perform them. Liza, a married woman of seventy-five, falls at least daily, can no longer drive, could not walk a block, can no longer crochet, read, or cook, and lives with chronic pain and rigidity.

SAMANTHA: Well, it's strange. Some people have it for years and others go downhill very quickly.

LIZA: I know. I wish I was like that.

SAMANTHA: Why do you say that?

LIZA: I am getting tired living like this. You still try to put on a nice front, though. Deep down I'd just soon be gone as [live like this].

Everett, who is almost ten years older than Liza, unmarried, takes more medications than Liza, falls weekly, and deals with frequent bouts of freezing, takes a far more optimistic view of his PD prognosis

> I can't see that I've had any progression. Yes, I take that back, I have had progression. I don't get up out of a chair very well. I have to think about it and get myself poised, and then sometimes it takes two or three shots at it to get up. It seems very dumb because you don't feel weak, it's just that you don't quite get it done. . . . Posture is a problem. And not all of the time. I can be walking along perfectly normal one day, the next day I'll get up [and my posture will be what] they call simian or ape-like. So you can stop and straighten yourself up and you can take about five steps and you're back in it again. It's just, it's really freaky. It looks like you oughta be able to say, "Now, straighten up!" you know. . . . I feel good. I notice a difference in stamina. I used to play three sets of tennis and wasn't particularly tired. And now I play one or maybe one and a half, and that walk back up from the tennis courts, that's a long walk anymore. That would be the big difference that I noticed: I don't have the stamina that I had three years ago.
>
> I've been a little stubborn. I haven't let go of anything much. Well, I've used it as an excuse maybe to get out of some jobs that I would have had to do before. I may turn down a job on a committee now. "I don't think I want to do that." And doctors have said, you know, "If it's at all stressful, just don't do it. You don't need to." And I've done a lot of that

kind of work. I feel like I've paid my rent. I'm not golfing well at all. I never was a great golfer, but I used to shoot in the forties and I have a hard time breaking fifty now. The same with the tennis. I'm about a step slower than I was a year ago. But I'm playing with old guys, and I can hold up my end of the game pretty much. . . . One thing that I've given up . . . I had an accident. I was driving and I went to sleep. It makes me a little nervous about driving now, and I don't drive long distances. I was driving [a] 325-mile drive and I got about 290 of it in when I had the accident. I hadn't had any problems about driving prior to that. I'm a little cautious now, and I drive shorter distances. Try to plan ahead as much as I can on the driving. . . .

I wish I didn't have it, but if you were to pick a disease, I'd sure take it in preference to cancer or something like that. Because it, in most cases, it doesn't keep you from living a pretty normal life. Now, obviously I'm one of the fortunate ones. It hasn't progressed very much. Because I have seen acquaintances of mine that have gotten it and been gone in three or four years. And really just gone downhill. Somebody says, "Well, you have such a good attitude about it." I don't think maybe the attitude has a lot to do with it. It makes it easier for me, that I can treat having the disease as not being all shook up about it, but I'm not sure that your attitude has much to do with how well you get along. I think you're lucky if you don't progress.

While Everett is more secure financially and more physically functional than Liza is, his impairments have not restricted him from doing the primary activities in which he finds meaning. In comparison, the things which shaped Liza's days—cooking for her family, visiting friends in the neighborhood, making gifts for grandchildren, doing puzzles, and reading the paper—have been severely constrained. Liza's scope of influence has been reduced to the family and friends that come to visit, and her day's activities to watching television.

The meaning of progression also depends in part on how it is measured. People measure progression by dividing the changes in their abilities from diagnosis to the present by the number of years that they've had PD. It is not an exact arithmetic. In Everett's case, even though he listed quite a few measures of decline, he did not really feel that his case had progressed. His declines have accumulated over fifteen years of having the disorder, and he would characterize himself as a "slow progressor." In contrast, Leroy would label himself a "fast progressor." In less than a decade he went from being somewhat athletic and active to presenting the archetypal stooped, shuffling PD posture. At sixty-nine, he recounts his progression: "Well, [during] the first three years, I don't [think there was much of a decline]. I mean, I still walked and my walk was mostly normal. I didn't worry about freezing up. I really didn't know what 'on and off'

meant. And the next three has been a steady deterioration. It's quite a difference now, between now and seven years ago when I went in. I couldn't possibly
jog. I walk. And I have a treadmill and I walk on that every day. But I tire very easily. So, in that respect, yeah, it's been a deterioration."

The prediction and assessment of progression and its temporal framework
was prominent in the minds of people I interviewed. They wondered, "What is
normal progression?" and "What can I expect?" as Leroy's remarks illustrate:

> I was just asking [my doctor] this last week: "Is there . . . a point at which
> everybody, at seven years, is about the same? Or does it vary a lot with
> people?" He thought it varied a lot with people, where you were. And so,
> as far as I compare myself, I think I must be about where you'd be
> expected to be. I don't think I'm worse off. I think you can do a lot with
> just the approach that you take yourself towards the disease. You can't do
> anything about having it. You can sit around and mope about it. But it
> won't do you any good. The only thing that you can control is the attitude
> that you've got, the way you approach it. Just stay busy and try and do
> things that you're really interested in. I think you can improve your out-
> look on it. Whether that does anything with the progression or not,
> I wouldn't have any idea. And I don't think that any of those doctors that I
> talk to would have any idea either, what controls the progression. But
> I would say that I am not any worse off than anybody else that has it.

This temporal piece of having PD and considering one's future with it is also
reflected in Lucille's story about telling people that she had PD. Lucille, in her
early seventies, said: "We went and told our minister right away. I didn't tell the
ladies at church. I told them once, and I don't think they believed me. I was
shaking one time and a lady says, 'What's with you?' And I said, 'I *told* you I had
PD.' And she said, 'Oh, you really do.' Some people think that once you are diagnosed with it you are going to [require] total care. I didn't think it would be
immediate, but I did think it would progress faster than it has. I really do all of
my activities of daily living."

People like Lucille, who had reconciled themselves to the unknowing, were
then faced with other people's beliefs about PD prognosis. Just as Harry's friends
had begun to decide for him what he was still able to do, choosing to invite him
only to events that they determined he was able to attend (see chapter 4),
Lucille's friends assumed that a PD diagnosis meant total disability.

Retired Lives or Retirement? Zen Masters and Master Planners

Retirement is an ongoing role, not a discrete event. Savishinsky's (2000) beau-
tiful study of the meanings of retirement shows us that ideas concerning older
age and aging contribute to people's adaptations to the end of work life. He

describes the rite of passage of the retirement ritual, consisting of informal rites (e.g., an office party), the gift, a guest list (to pay "final respects"), travel plans, and the rhetoric and fantasy regarding the freedoms of a work-free life. Retirement is seen as a period in life designed for relaxation, leisure activities, and travel. Ironically, despite this freedom from schedules, retirement is something that many Americans plan for. Savishinsky characterizes two types of retirement planners—Zen masters and master planners. Zen masters are elders who allow retirement to happen to them, who if they make plans do so based on their current desires and abilities. In contrast, master planners work to establish a sense of mastery over their retirement, planning their activities and focusing on potentialities, be they somatic or economic.

The study participants with whom I worked are little different. Some had planned doing extensive travel, attending senior college, learning a new language, or remodeling their kitchens. Others simply anticipated having more time to do the things they already enjoyed; they did not require a schedule to accomplish their retirement plan. Of course, those diagnosed at a younger age had already envisioned their retirements as PD patients and had adjusted their plans accordingly. Those who were diagnosed after retirement were dismayed by the changes they had to make. When relating their retirement aspirations to me they explained, "Well, I didn't *plan* to get PD." One seventy-seven-year-old caretaker was grateful for the good years in retirement, before the disease progressed:

> I knew we had quite a few years of productivity, you know, really. And it is treatable, especially today. There are so many medications. And he has done very well on his medications. It's just been in the, what, latter few years where you have so much freezing and stuff. Maybe I accepted it because I knew what was in store down the road, having taken care of so many people I know. It can either be a very progressive, fast disease, which I have seen in different ones that have been diagnosed at the same time he was. Or it can be a slow thing. And for him its just kind of a slow process. . . . We were able to still travel. We don't do as much now. I do most of the driving. . . . It does put a damper on a lot of things. You don't do all of the things that you normally thought you would do in retirement years. It's a good thing we started when we did.

For some families PD required a slower, less ambitious pace. Travel plans were simplified, pared down, and abandoned. Hobbies that required fine motor skills and exertion were given up. And PD was to blame. Obviously, PD's effect on the body, wallet, and mental health can contribute to a reduction in social engagement or leisure activity, but the normal aging process can do this, too. Older adults may tire more easily and develop muscle stiffness or delayed reaction times, all of which could impact a golf swing or crocheted stitch. But no one I spoke with ever blamed old age for their relinquishment of retirement activities—PD was the condition placed on retirement plans. Here, PD obscures the effects of aging and serves as a conduit to transition to new roles in later life—for both sufferers and caregivers.

Clyde, who at sixty-two years old was still working full-time, exemplifies the Zen master approach to retirement.

CLYDE: Mine has progressed slowly. [I plan to retire] in a couple of years. Well, I will probably get drunk and chase young girls around. [laughs] No. We have a small farm now, we've got about twenty acres, and I just bought a larger farm, about two hundred acres. We are going to move there in about two years. I will have plenty of stuff to keep me busy. I will be a "retired farmer farmer." We got a lot of brush to clear, fences to build. I mean, I was raised on a farm and I want to go back to a farm.

SAMANTHA: What do you think about moving to a more isolated area and bigger piece of land when you have a progressive condition? Does that enter in your decision?

CLYDE: Yeah. It does. My wife and I have talked about that. I guess, you know, you've heard the expression of, "He just keeps planting trees"? Well, I am just going to keep planting trees, what the heck. I don't want to sit here and say, "All right, we've got to start circling our wagons," because at some point in my life I might not be functional. I'm going to keep going. If at some point in my life I become nonfunctional, then I guess we will deal with that.

Clyde's outlook on retirement differed greatly from that of Lillian, a retired woman who at seventy-two was planning ahead in case she became less functional.

I have decided that these steps [in her townhouse] are getting the best of me. There are sixteen steps. I have started looking for either another townhouse that is all on one floor or an apartment building that might have elevators or something like that. The last couple of weeks I have spent a lot of time doing that. . . . It is just that I had a couple of near-mishaps going up the steps with my hands full. I decided that it was time. The fellow who takes care of finances and so forth for me is also going to be the one who has to take care of me when I become more disabled—if I become more disabled. I had a talk with him and he said, "Well, I was wondering when that day would come. I just didn't think it would be this soon. I am glad that you are making the decision yourself." . . . I don't want anybody to have to come in and say, "Lillian, you've got to move tomorrow. And this is where you are going." Not if I still have any faculties of my own, at least. [laughs] I want to have some say on that.

While Lillian's outlook may differ in part due to her retiree status, she and Clyde were virtually matched for symptoms, medication use, and overall function. Perhaps more important was Lillian's marital status. Whereas Clyde could look to his wife and children for support, Lillian had never married, had no children, and her living family was more disabled than she. In another sense, though, we can see that in response to an unpredictable condition, some people elect to accept their lack of control and others feel compelled to exert what control they feel they possess.

The difference between Zen masters and master planners is evident in people's decisions to stop driving and scale back travel plans. A few months prior to my fieldwork, an unusual automobile accident in California made front-page news across the country. An older man had driven his car into a crowded farmer's market, killing eight bystanders and injuring more than a dozen (LeDuff 2003). I was teaching an introductory course in aging studies at the time, and I was eager to hear my students' reviews of the media coverage. All but one student was between the ages of nineteen and twenty-two years old. They were pursuing a variety of degrees, including nursing, business, accounting, creative writing, and social work. All but the lone nontraditional student, a middle-aged social work major, argued for age-limited driver's licenses or mandatory testing of older drivers. I was disappointed. After weeks of discussing age discrimination and stereotypes, the deeply embedded biases against older adult drivers held fast. The heated national debate visited these issues but thankfully subsided after accomplishing little to nothing. Invariably, when the topic was raised in a support group meeting, PD patients became defensive or argumentative, and caregivers fell quiet.

PD sufferers exchanged numerous stories of discrimination and bureaucracy relating to the Department of Motor Vehicles (DMV). If the DMV clerk was aware of your disease status, she would require you to obtain a physician's consent in order for you to renew your license. This consent involved another trip to the doctor's office, a series of lengthy forms, and a second trip to the DMV. Depending on the physician's assessment, PD patients may also be required to take another road test. In light of this, many strategies for "beating the system" circulated at support group meetings. Sufferers encouraged each other to renew their licenses during their peak medication period and to utilize their medication window to its fullest extent. In other words, it doesn't make sense to go when you are feeling tired or are nearing the next medication time. Some people advised taking extra medication to ensure full function during a stressful time. Some identified certain DMV staff known to be more attentive or particular than others, so that these staff persons could be avoided. Because stress and crowds can exacerbate tremor and freezing, some suggested, PD sufferers should avoid going to the DMV on a Monday or Friday because the office was less busy midweek. Following this logic, others recommended that people go to suburban or rural test centers, so that if they had to take a road test, the setting would be less congested and stressful. Very few people openly advocated lying and denying that one had PD when questioned, but subtle deception was an important strategy. Elders advised each other to leave their walkers and canes in the car to avoid incrimination and to downplay their tremor when asked by saying, "Oh, that's nothing," or "An old war injury." Another deception involved redirecting blame for incorrect test answers: If someone made a mistake on the vision or written exam, they could blame it on the examiner by accusing them of asking a different question. The test taker could then request permission to repeat the test again.

When pressed, a majority recognized that they wouldn't be able to drive indefinitely, but few people could identify their personal criterion for deciding that it was time to stop driving. The licenses of the Zen masters in the group would have to be pried out of their hands. The mobility that cars and licenses promised, even for someone who rarely drove, gained importance because PD had decreased their physical mobility. The lack of ambulatory skill makes other forms of mobility important. This is doubly so for those elders who continued to reside in rural areas. Cars were the only means by which they could access groceries, health care, and social activities. However, the risk of driving at all once labeled with PD encouraged a few of the master-planner types to give up driving while they were still quite competent at it. This minority explained to me that should they ever be involved in a motor vehicle accident, no matter who or what was at fault, they would surely be blamed because they were twice at fault—they were old and they had PD. Again, in the face of uncertainty, master planners choose to find ways to exert control over their lives.

On a related issue, snowbirds—Iowans who rode out the state's six months of cold and ice down in sunny Arizona and Texas—had to make decisions about the continued viability of their lifestyle. The three- to four-day drive, the responsibility and cost of maintaining two homes, the work involved in packing and preparing each place for extended vacancies, and the great geographic distance between familiar doctors—all over time grow in importance as deciding factors. Even though virtually all snowbirds find economic incentive in purchasing their medications at a low cost in Mexico, the overall cost of the snowbird lifestyle was high. Zen masters like Ruby, who was seventy-eight, focused on the positive aspects of living in the Southwest, and their narratives stressed the social outlets available to them there:

> We hope [to stay in our home]. It's really cheaper than going to a town house or anything like that. I don't think [my husband would] be happy in a town house. He likes to do his yard. I hope we can stay for quite a while. He's down there [in the basement] most of the time; he's got projects going. He will pick up things and put them back together, you know. Paint them and fix them all up and then sell them in his yard sale. In the wintertime we go out to Arizona, and he keeps busy out there all of the time, too. It's kind of funny to see all of these older people in the campgrounds, riding bicycles and playing baseball. . . . It's not funny; it's just

different from here. Here you don't see people our age riding bicycles around the street and running around playing baseball. And tennis and shuffleboard. It's a different life altogether. When you get home, why it's kind of boring for a couple months. Not really boring, just different.

Master planners, by contrast, emphasize the importance of making choices while they are still available, as this exchange between Russell, seventy-nine, and his wife implies:

SAMANTHA: Are you planning on continuing to go down to Arizona?

CAREGIVER: Well, the last few years I've wanted to sell it, but he doesn't want to. . . .

RUSSELL: This is her talk. Let me put it this way. This is *her* talk. We haven't had an agreement on this yet.

CAREGIVER: Of course not. He won't sell. I said, "Well one of us is going to get stuck with it." I don't want that.

Despite having dealt with two medical crises during their most recent trip south, Russell is adamant that they not sell their Arizona home. His wife, a master planner, disagrees. She stresses the importance of making a decision before the option is taken away, and before she may be forced to make the decision alone.

Everyone that I met hoped to live in their current residence for the remainder of their lives, and no one discussed long-term care options in a positive light. Yet, even over the relatively short span of fifteen months, the effects of PD progression compelled people to rethink their plans. At the outset of the project everyone lived in private residences, whether suburban spilt levels, mobile homes, or apartments. Toward the end of my fieldwork at least two dozen households had relocated into a continuous care or other long-term care facility. Of course, much of the impetus for these moves came directly from PD, but other important factors included pressure from adult children and service availability. Three large continuous care facilities opened up within the last twelve months of my field research, making such services available for the first time in two communities.

People who chose not to move were not necessarily less impaired, but may have had socioeconomic constraints. Anecdotal evidence from field observations suggested that economic responsibility for adult children, low educational attainment, and lower income were barriers to relocation. A few of these people spoke of nursing homes as inevitable in their future and made dark suggestions that nursing homes would be the place where their battle with PD was lost.

Eva, at eighty-four, remarked that she'd prefer death to living in a state of impairment that required nursing home care.

EVA: [When I was first diagnosed,] I thought, "Well, there really should be something that could cure that." But there hasn't been, I guess. [laughs]

SAMANTHA: Well, there is one way out, but lets hope it's a long time before you get there.

EVA: Oh, you mean the "final step"? [laughs] If I can't take care of myself and I can't be civil to people, I don't want to be gross, but I am ready to go if that's it. But, I don't want to have to lay in bed and be fed and stuff.

SAMANTHA: No one wants to picture the end of their lives like that.

EVA: My sister keeps telling me, "Well, yours doesn't advance very fast." She had taken care of people with PD and she says, "You've got a long, long ways to go." But it is so dreadful when it gets so bad. I keep that in the back of my mind. If there is anything I can do to stop it coming to get me.

Eva's sentiments echoed Helen's, who late in the study had two parents with PD. Helen's father died in a long-term care center. She described the indignities he experienced during his stay and how he pleaded with her to take him home for care. Helen was determined to avoid a long-term care facility herself and took steps toward preserving her independence. As described earlier, she and her husband downsized their residence from a large sprawling suburban home to a small, one-story town house with no outdoor responsibilities. Yet, despite her plans, about a year after our interview Helen suffered a sudden and severe decline. She was hospitalized and then institutionalized. I spoke to her on the telephone, and she sobbed that she didn't want to speak to me from the nursing home, that she didn't want me to see her in this condition, and that she was going to go back home soon. Helen died a few weeks later.

Progression or Aging?

Aging is a social process of transformation. People age into new caregiving roles (from child rearing to spousal care and grandparenting), occupations (from paid to leisure and volunteer), and somatic experiences (from growth to slowed healing and potential decline). As Savishinsky's (2000) work describes, older Americans approach this transformation in different ways, with some striving to establish plans and schedules which will accommodate change, and others who desire to live out their remaining years as an extension of their life course narrative, without substantive agendas. Both groups seek to achieve a sense of mastery over lives made uncertain by a progressive disorder, but they do it differently. Zen masters focus on aspects of their lives which give them joy and satisfaction in the present moment, whereas master planners focus on extending their life satisfaction by planning for potential losses. These approaches are complicated when a condition such as PD arises. Not only does PD function as a set of interrelated somatic and social constraints on lived experience, but also it works to alter elders' embodiment of age relative to their current chronological age.

Aging and PD alike compel many people to make plans for having reduced capacities. PD is a condition overlaid on these processes. PD sufferers in their sixties described feeling old before their time, as if their aging had been accelerated. Much of this has to do with the somatic experience, but it extends to their retirement decisions as well. Young-old PD sufferers are drawn into making decisions about relocating, financial security, insurance, and reduced travel plans at an earlier age than they expected or than seems normal. The middle-old group, whose aging is mediated by PD, viewed progression as a dialectic between aging and PD. They attributed changes in their retirement plans and expectations to aging and PD equally, recognizing the impossibility of separating the two. Yet the oldest-old group rarely spoke of age affecting their retirement decisions at all. Rather, those for whom PD obscures normal aging attributed every limitation on their plans to the diagnosis. Whereas young-old people prematurely aged and the middle old felt conflicted about aging and PD, the oldest old almost denied aging as a factor in their lives.

The variability of PD progression is integral to sufferers' retirement decisions and predisposition toward becoming master planners or Zen masters. PD sufferers contend with unpredictability every day, asking themselves questions like: Will my medications work well today? Will I be able to stay awake during the banquet speeches tonight? Will my hands work the way that I want them to today? Will this be a good day or a bad day? Freezing and wearing off are daily and hourly reminders that one's sense of control and self-efficacy are transitory and cannot be relied upon. In this context, rate of progression becomes an almost nonsensical issue. Not only may someone's case of PD change in one month, one year, or five years, but the scope of those changes directs what sorts of interventions or accommodations will be required. Sufferers with predominantly cognitive but slow-progressing PD may be pushed toward institutional care much more rapidly than others who have more quickly advancing mobility-focused cases. The importance of particular somatic changes is a product of identity development over someone's life course. PD sufferers may dread the loss of a particular ability, but their inability to predict whether they will experience that loss, and when, makes it difficult to determine what might be reasonable accommodations to prepare.

That so many of the PD sufferers relocated toward the end of my fifteen-month study may seem unsurprising to most people, who might assume that PD's progressive nature compels people to plan for loss. Yet, in the context of rural Iowa, this is a relatively new approach to later life's needs. While one man explained to me that this is "about the age when you begin to expect things to happen," another countered, "While I knew the Parkinson's was going to slow me down somewhat, I thought that by keeping in shape and by keeping exercising

I could do many of the things that we had hoped to do. But it hasn't turned out that way. And, as [my wife] often says, it's wonderful that we did what we wanted when we were able to. I don't have any regrets about any of the trips that we have taken or the hiking that we have done, but I sure hope to do a lot more of it. It's again, almost every day in the mail I get some kind of brochure for travel of some kind, and now I just hardly look at them. I just put them into the recycle bin and forget about them, I guess. It has been a blow."

These conflicting attitudes toward the inevitability of loss both in later life and in the context of PD frame the range of beliefs concerning planning for accommodation. In communities where independence and self-reliance are integral components of moral and cultural fiber, planning for loss seems to run counter to the humility and grace with which Iowan elders approach their impairments. Rather than viewing themselves as sick people with a disease in need of treatment, elder PD sufferers consider themselves relatively healthy, except for this aggravating condition of PD—a condition they try to get along with as best they can, day by day, without fanfare.

8

Changing Bodies, Changing Roles

Introduction: Living Apart from Your Spouse

Audrey invited me to meet her at her new apartment, located just a few minutes' drive from the nursing home where her husband, Glen, now resided. When she answered the door, I was struck by how young she looked. At only sixty years old she has already had to make decisions often thought of as end-of-life planning. While her husband was ten years her senior and not actively dying, his PD had progressed until she could no longer sleep for more than several hours at a time without waking up worried that he might be endangering himself or her.

We sat across from one another at a small kitchen table and spent the next two hours talking about her life with Glen and the strange marriage one has when forced to live apart from one's spouse. About ten years ago, Glen began to complain that his legs felt "funny," as if they weighed a hundred pounds and were made of cement. He started to have trouble walking, and both he and Audrey suspected PD. Even though they had an inkling of what it was, it took months and visits to two neurologists to arrive at a diagnosis. At the time, they viewed the PD diagnosis as a resolution, Audrey says. "When he first got the diagnosis it wasn't a bad thing. The realization of what is to come is not there yet. You kind of deny it. Actually, for about four years we didn't really have a whole lot of trouble. He had the shaking. And he took the medicine and that kind of thing. There wasn't too much trouble, but then after about four years of that he started getting worse. And the last four years have been a real struggle for him."

For four years carbidopa-levodopa and an antidepressant controlled Glen's symptoms enough that he was able to continue his work as a clergyman. Then, falling became a daily, then an hourly occurrence, and it was nerve-wracking to watch him walk across a room. Glen's mobility impairments and his increasing instability led him to give up driving, Audrey says. "My husband has made it very easy for me by declaring, 'Take my car keys and don't give them back to me.'

He realized he shouldn't be driving anymore. He has also said that he didn't
want me to be burdened with him. I never felt like I was burdened with him. It
was always him thinking he was a burden."

At that point Audrey decided that they should move from their home to a
more accessible apartment with fewer responsibilities. She was not yet sixty, but
Glen's age qualified them for an assisted-living facility. Audrey appreciated the
benefits such housing offered Glen, but she often felt out of place, being the
youngest and most able-bodied person in the community. Her oldest neighbor
was ninety-seven and she had to stretch to find things in common with people
her husband's age or older.

It was only a year later when Audrey herself needed medical attention and
required inpatient surgery. During her recovery period, she caught up on some
much-needed rest while Glen was cared for in a nursing home. When Audrey
was ready to bring Glen back home, his physician informed her that Glen might
be better cared for in a facility setting. She describes that time:

> When the diagnosis did come back that he had severe dementia, we
> knew that he had to be in a safer place. He was getting up five, six, seven
> times a night. I would have to get up with him and I was not getting any
> sleep. I was getting jumpy, because every noise I heard I thought it was
> him getting up. He also became incontinent during that time. It just kind
> of went downhill real fast. . . . All of these changes all came at once. It was
> hard, I'm sure, on his body, to get through all of those medical changes.
> Plus trying to accept being in a nursing home, which is not an easy thing
> to do when you think that you are going to live there for ten years—
> although I have been told that it won't be that long.

However, having made the decision to move Glen to the nursing home, Audrey
was faced with having to move again herself. She was too young to qualify for an
apartment in the assisted-living community. Her worries were amplified by
their increasing financial outlays. While they still had the proceeds from the
sale of their home, they were paying about $2,400 a month for rent and roughly
$800 for Glen's PD medications. Audrey had paid for Glen's first nursing home
stay out of pocket. During that time the cost of his medications alone topped
$2,000. She was currently working to get him enrolled in Medicaid, which
meant going through a complicated process of dividing their joint assets and
then spending down Glen's account to a $2,000 balance. Once she accom-
plished that, he would be eligible for Medicaid and she would have retained the
maximum amount of their estate to take care of her during her retirement.
When we talked, Audrey and Glen were living off their savings, and she was
unsure how much they owed for Glen's medical expenses. Audrey's lack of
knowledge about the extent of their debts and about her ability to continue to
maintain her standard of living weighed heavily on her mind.

The recent moves and Glen's deteriorating cognitive health have introduced stressors into what was a collegial and warm marriage. Glen is alert enough at times to recognize that he can no longer serve the faith community as a clergyman, but he misses this important aspect of his life. He insists that people refer to him as "doctor," commensurate with his PhD in divinity. As Audrey told me, "He wants people to know that he was somebody." And yet he is no longer the person that she married. Not only is she living apart from her husband, but also at times he is almost unrecognizable. Audrey struggles to interpret his changing personality and his childlike behavior and fights to resist feeling that she has abandoned her husband. At the same time, Audrey recognizes that she now has some time to recuperate from years of physically and mentally demanding caregiving.

Audrey spoke at length about her adjustment process:

I am still working on it. It's very sad to have your mate not living with you. This is the first time in years and years that I have lived alone. . . . And now I am having to live alone and there is a lot of quiet time [to wonder,] "Gee, what am I going to do with my life now?" I am a pastor's wife, but still things do bother you. Faithwise, you question, "Why does a man of God have to have something so horrific? Somebody who has dedicated his whole life to God and this is the reward he gets here on earth?" [laughs] . . . Living with elderly people and seeing the different people around me and how they suffer and how life is for them at this time makes me almost hate to get old. I am old, but to get *older*, you know. . . .

Illness can really take its toll, not only physically but emotionally and spiritually, on a person. My faith has helped me get through all of it. The thing I miss the most is a sense of joy in living. When you think you have to eat alone and you have to go everywhere alone, . . . it's just . . . you are married, but you don't have a mate living with you. It's just a tough, tough thing to go through. I guess what I want to say is that it is sad to see somebody that you love decline and see something daily, almost, happening in their life. And see the pain in their eyes because they know that this is happening.

My husband is one of these that doesn't want me to have to suffer or him be a burden to me. Now, the day that I took him from one nursing home to the other, I was feeling so guilty that I had to give up taking care of him. I told him. I said, "Please forgive me for putting you in a nursing home." He didn't respond to me. And so I said to him, "Honey, did you hear what I said?" And he said, "Well, I've been thinking. And that's something you don't need to ask forgiveness for." So if I hadn't said my feelings, I would have had that guilt, always. And just like that it lifted.

After our interview, Audrey and I drove over to the nursing home to visit Glen. While I had never been to this facility before, it felt familiar nonetheless—the long, spare hallways decorated in pastel greens, the scent of potpourri, urine, and antiseptic, and a blaring television with several wheelchair-bound elders parked in front of it. It was a place where no one *planned* to move and a place that very few people left alive. We arrived to find Glen lying in bed watching his small television set at a high volume. Audrey introduced us and then left the room so that we could talk a while. Glen treated me as a student and seemed happy to answer my short, directed questions. He explained that he would prefer not to live there, but that he knew he had to. He spoke of his wife lovingly. She took good care of him, he told me. And as it often does in nursing homes, time slowed to a creep. We spoke for about thirty minutes, but when we parted I felt that I had been there for hours. Despite his shaking arms and legs, his inability to sit up on his own or feed himself, Glen was having a good day, it seemed. He knew Audrey, and he could carry on a conversation. He was "somebody," if only for a brief time.

Audrey and I regrouped and went to dinner together. While she at times felt that her life was on hold, we discussed her social life and her eagerness to get out and see people again. Glen's move to the nursing home freed up a little bit of her time. She visited him at least once a day for a few hours, but now she could sleep through the night without having to keep one eye open to watch for Glen's safety. Audrey shared her sense of anticipation with me at the possibility for something new to happen—a new friendship, a new hobby, some time for her to get caught up on correspondence. At the same time, she was undergoing treatment for her own depression and feeling chronic sorrow for both her husband, who used to be "somebody," and his daily reconfiguring of who he was at that moment.

PD Caregiving: Stress, Gain, and Life Transitions

PD sufferers' identity and their sense of autonomy, privacy, and personal space adapt to the disorder's progressive demands on the body. However isolated these adaptations may make PD sufferers feel, they do not make such changes alone: Spouses must also adapt. The balance between doing and receiving in the daily equilibrium of a household changes in response to PD sufferers' impairments. These adaptations are often called "caregiving," and they reflect long-lived marital tensions as well as caregiver and PD sufferer notions of what it means to grow older. These changes are easy to see in Glen and Audrey's case, but even in less advanced cases, PD inextricably shapes husbands' and wives' interactions with one another. PD sufferers and caregivers both find that they must relax their definition of their partners' role in order to maintain the integrity of their relationship. Certainly, some married couples maintained their prescribed gender and marital roles and their division of household labor. But a majority of households lived somewhere in between their traditional roles and "living apart." An eighty-year-old caregiver talked about her feelings for her husband with PD: "I must confess that I did not realize that this disease has an impact on everything. It affects everything in a relationship, and it is so difficult to see the person you love experience all these changes and all you can do is be there for them and be very supportive. . . . This is very difficult to deal with. The person you love and have lived with for fifty years plus changes before your eyes. I have difficulty dealing with the fact that he will not return to the person I have known and loved. I try to keep fighting for him and don't always succeed."

Much research on caregiving in PD focuses upon the impact of caregiving activities on caregivers' health and well-being. Disease severity and longevity negatively influence caregiver health (Berry and Murphy 1995; Birgersson and Edberg 2004; Lindgren 1996; McRae, Sherry, and Roper 1999; Wallhagan and Brod 1997). A caregiver's burden increases as the sufferer's management of PD symptoms decreases (Edwards 2002). PD sufferer depression is associated with caregiver depression (Caap-Ahlgren, Lannerheim, and Dehlin 2002; Fernandez et al. 2001). The decline of a sufferer's health may increase the demands on a caregiver's time, socially isolating them (McRae, Sherry, and Roper 1999). Compared to noncaregiving elders of similar age, caregivers are less likely to have had a vacation or be able to leave the house to socialize with friends (O'Reilly et al. 1996). PD caregivers "are providing an inordinate amount of health care services, on a daily basis, and at great cost to their own welfare" (Berry and Murphy 1995). These caregivers perform strenuous, tedious, and "dirty" work. They assist their spouses with transferring to bed, chairs, or toilets, dressing, managing medications, or bathing. In general, the frequency and intensity of caregiving demands increase as PD progresses. The largest components of family burden are informal caregiving and wages lost due to time spent caregiving (Whettan-Goldstein et al. 1997).

Across disorders, caregivers commonly report feelings of shame, guilt, low self-esteem, anxiety, frustration, and stress (Bond, Clark, and Davies 2003). PD caregivers report these emotions, but the disorder has its own unique challenges. PD's unpredictability means that caregivers must be vigilant to continuously adjust their level of care in response to their partners' immediate abilities (Berry and Murphy 1995; O'Reilly et al. 1996). The caregiver may be the spouse's sole social outlet, especially when speech problems render the partner's voice only intimately intelligible. McRae, Sherry, and Roper's (1999) study of the contributors to PD caregiver stress assessed the degree of significance among sources of strain. Least significant were caregivers' concerns about what others might think of their household or their spouse. The most stressful aspects of caregiving were fear of the future, anxiety, social isolation, and fatigue.

Lindgren's work on chronic sorrow is also illustrative. Chronic sorrow is the cyclical experience of "grief from continual losses over the trajectory of an illness or disability" and periods of calm. In her mixed methods study of PD caregivers, chronic sorrow was common but not universal. Sorrow episodes were stimulated by falls and signs of disease progression (1996, 351). Lyons et al. (2004) studied a group of couples for ten years and found that caregiver pessimism at the outset of the study is a predictor of poor future health of caregivers, while caregiver optimism is associated with better health and lower perceived impact. A phenomenological study by Birgersson and Edberg (2004) compared PD sufferers' and caregivers' appraisal of social and instrumental support. They described PD sufferers as being "in the light of support": Even though they did not receive enough information regarding their condition, they continued to assess their social support positively. In contrast, caregivers were "in the shade" of support, lacking the psychosocial resources to positively engage in their roles and maintain their health.

Many studies of PD and other caregiving situations conceptualize the role as a burden, stress, or strain. Kramer ventures that this terminology may inadvertently cast caregiving in a negative light and emphasizes the importance of explicating caregiving's multidimensional nature. Relatively less studied are how caregiver gains—the benefits caregivers can receive from this role—can help to predict positive outcomes. Gains can be conceptualized as discrete activities, such as the care receiver's expressions of gratitude, or as a positive appraisal of caregiving as a role. Bond, Clark, and Davies (2003) integrate the stresses and gains within their life transition model. This conceptualization of caregiving acknowledges the often profound adjustment that caregivers make to accommodate their partners' needs, as the comments of this eighty-seven-year-old caregiver I spoke with reveal: "Of course it has made a big difference in my schedule. I have had to give up attending some organizations I enjoyed, and much around the home is left undone. But the rewards are plentiful. I have my husband around much more, and we enjoy the times when we are going and coming from appointments whenever we can get out. And I have a bigger purpose besides my home and my interests—to do for him what he can no longer do."

How stressful caregiving is depends upon the individual caregiver's valuation of the role (O'Reilly et al. 1996), and a life transitions approach allows us to examine caregiving as an embodied experience.

Iowa PD Caregivers

Iowa caregivers experience the physical and emotional stresses and gains reported in academic literature. Caregivers aged sixty-five and older scored below the fiftieth percentile on all RAND MOS scales. They also scored significantly lower than the general population overall on the bodily pain and general health scores. When compared to a standardized population of the same age and gender, female caregivers fared significantly more poorly than did males. In addition, caregivers' assessment of the intensity and frequency of their caregiving was higher than that of their spouses. Caregivers were significantly more likely to report that they provided transportation, managed their spouse's medications and appointments, and performed the laundry, financial, and housekeeping tasks. When caregiver and sufferer reports were compared by gender, male caregivers' reports were not significantly higher than those of their spouses for paying bills, preparing meals, or keeping appointments and female caregivers' reports were not higher than those of their husbands for shopping, picking up around the house, or doing the laundry. These gender differences likely reflect couples' longstanding household division of labor.

Formal services are admittedly scant in much of the geographic area in which I conducted fieldwork, but even families who resided in suburban areas with extensive service networks seldom used them. Roughly 10 percent of questionnaire respondents used housekeeping services, just over 5 percent used a congregate meal site or Meals on Wheels, and only a handful used other available services such as a lifeline emergency call service, home health nurse, telephone assurance program, adult day care, respite care, or elderly case management.

I conducted several interviews with caregivers for very disabled sufferers, such as the one with Audrey, but most of my understanding of caregiving is drawn from in-home observations and caregivers' handwritten responses to these open-ended questionnaire items:

In what ways, if any, has your loved one's Parkinson's affected your relationship with them?

Please take a moment to comment on how Parkinson's has impacted your day-to-day activities and the things you enjoy spending time doing.

Does your role as a caregiver of someone with Parkinson's present any special challenges or rewards?

Do you feel that your family has had to change its retirement plans because of what Parkinson's may bring? If so, what kinds of changes has your family made?

Most often, my ethnographic gaze was trained upon the bodies of PD sufferers as they worked to maintain their identity in the face of unpredictable impairments. The meaning of their bodies and how aging comes to be embodied is understood in the spaces where the body fails to meet its ideal—the social space where caregivers reside. Caregivers seemed at times to be on the periphery of the project, always there to share their insights or to help their spouse into a chair, but rarely at the center. Accordingly, I structure my discussion of caregiving in relational terms. In the caregiving dialectic, PD's effect on the meaning of aging is both a product of long-lived marital relationships and cocreated by couples in the moment.

Cooperative Efforts to Care for Uncooperative Bodies

PD can create a dramatically uncooperative and unattractive body. On the outside, PD can cause oily skin, incontinence, flaking scalp, heavy sweating, drooling, an expressionless face, trembling hands, or jerky, unruly limbs. On the inside, PD can cause swallowing and choking problems, shakiness, hallucinations, depression, anxiety, and constipation. Such changes are sources of embarrassment to PD sufferers, whose feelings of helplessness and frustration increase when their spouses become intimate in the devolving language of bodily fluids, limitations, and chronic pain.

Bodily fluids have been a rich source of ethnographic theory because they are invested with beliefs concerning pollution and social status (Douglas 1966; Jervis 2001). PD sufferers are embarrassed by their lack of control over their unruly bodily fluids. Their shame causes them to wait until the last minute to request help with what they feel are infantilizing chores. Caregivers reported that they have to become prognosticators; they must divine the needs of their spouses because their spouses won't admit a need for help, and they want to avoid incontinence events rather than spend time cleaning them up. Although caregivers recognized their partners' inability to control their bladder, a few caregivers saw their partners' drooling as intentional and controllable. One caregiver admitted that her husband's drooling disgusted her, and she was constantly reminding him to close his mouth. Her embarrassment at his drooling in public was palpable; she was frustrated with him: "Why can't he do this one thing for me?" When drooling came up in a support group meeting conversation, sufferers focused on strategies to remind themselves to swallow (such as sucking on hard candy). One man said, "Who cares? The slobbering is the least of my problems." But for Ethel, a sixty-year-old woman who retired early because of her PD symptoms, the embarrassment was manifest: "[I am bothered by] the stiffness in my legs and my arms and this slobbering. On a good day—I don't really ever have a good day. I always hurt. I always slobber. He put me on some medicine and that has helped some, but not enough."

Another symptom for which caregivers' assessment of control was not consistent with sufferers' efforts to mitigate expression was public dining. Tremor, dyskinesia, rigidity, and slowness work against the niceties of public dining. Some sufferers tried to circumvent spilling, slobbering, or loud eating by having their spouse cut their food up for them, tucking a napkin into their shirt as for a child, ordering their soup in a mug to be drunk rather than spooned, or ordering foods that were acceptable to eat with one's hands. As these comments show, the effort invested in polite behavior does not always translate into the hoped-for social norm. Henry, an eighty-two-year-old PD sufferer:

> After this morning, I'd say getting dressed is the biggest headache. It takes me a long time to get dressed. Especially when I have to put on something that looks halfway decent. Otherwise I can slip into a pair of

shorts or something and it doesn't take long. If I have to get *dressed*, it takes a bit longer. That, I would have to say, is the most difficult thing. Eating is difficult, but I manage to get by by shoveling it into my mouth. That's about what it amounts to—to keep it from spilling off of the spoon, you have to get it to your mouth pretty fast.

And a seventy-six-year-old caregiver:

My husband is physically very able. I often wonder if he has PD. However, his gait is different, his speech is very low and run together, he cannot remember to do things. His eating habits have deteriorated—he scoops his food. He stares at me often. He still completes all of the raking, mowing, repairs, gardening, et cetera, that he did before.

Caregivers confided that they were repulsed by their partners' eating habits and often embarrassed to watch them try to eat in public. The lack of motor control and the efforts sufferers made to retain dignity sometimes undermined their goals—wives chastised husbands for slurping loudly, shoveling their food into their mouths, or wearing their napkin on their chest. This disconnect may have increased the shame sufferers experienced as they did their best to perform under the constraints given.

Bodily fluids carry an enormous amount of psychological weight, but sufferers' bodies themselves contribute to physical strain on caregiver's bodies. I observed this firsthand on a visit to Martha and Joe's farmhouse. Joe is in his seventies and had to retire early because of his deteriorating concentration. Martha was about ten years younger than Joe and left her job to care for him full-time. As Joe's impairments increased, their cozy, sunny home presented accessibility barriers. Martha had a ramp installed outside the front door and grab bars installed in the bathroom. She moved their belongings down to the first-floor bedroom, and they mainly live in this part of the house. Joe can no longer climb stairs and must have a supporting arm or railing to walk safely. Martha has become a light sleeper in response to Joe's nighttime wandering. She has to make sure that he does not try to get out of bed by himself because he will fall and she has a hard time picking him up off the floor. Many caregivers live in fear that their partner will fall. Falls cause injuries and falls mean heavy lifting for the spouse or, worse yet, a call for emergency responder assistance and the medical cascade that entails.

While I was visiting one afternoon, Joe fell asleep in an armchair. Martha and I talked for several hours about her changing life and then we decided to break for dinner. She reached over to wake Joe and realized that he had had an incontinence episode. She sighed heavily. Without ado, she gently woke him up, reached her arms around him, and pulled him to stand. Joe was a foot taller, perhaps fifty pounds heavier, and had very little muscle tone or coordination.

Somehow Martha managed to help him upright and assisted his shuffling over to their bedroom. She helped him sit on the edge of the bed, she lifted his legs up onto the bed, and then she changed his clothes. This routine occurred several times a day, when Joe is incontinent, has to use the bathroom, or needs to bathe.

Sufferers and caregivers both are discouraged by sufferers' physical limitations. Caregivers stay home more often than they would like since they are afraid to leave their partners alone, and sometimes because going out is just too much trouble. It takes too long to wait for their spouse to get dressed (buttons, sleeves, zippers), go to the bathroom (zipper, throw rugs, sitting down, getting back up, constipation, adult diapers), get into the car (freezing, slowness, stiffness), and get out of the car. Some caregivers resent having to leave extra early to get anywhere on time, and having to slow themselves down to accommodate their partner's pace. Sometimes caregivers prefer to do all the household errands alone in order to complete them more efficiently and to have a few moments to themselves. With the exception of the snowbirds, retirees abandoned their lengthy travel rosters in deference to the physical limitations, economic shortfalls, and medication management that accompany PD. Caregivers try to limit their spouse's driving, may enlist the authority of a physician in revoking their partner's license, or simply take over all the driving. Sufferers object when their caregivers rush them, which worsens their tremor and freezing episodes. They dislike it when their partners automatically do things for them such as buttoning their shirt or helping them into the bathroom. These acts remind sufferers of their impairments and make them feel old. They generally prefer to do things on their own; self-sufficiency maintains dignity and, as one woman asserted, "You have to use it or lose it!"

Medication management emerged as another meaning-laden aspect of caregiving. Social activities may need to be organized around peak medication times, limiting couples' participation and travel. Caregivers become dispensaries, and one man explained that he felt like a prison warden. They were constantly asking their spouses if they had taken their medicines, reminding them to take them, picking medicine up at the pharmacy, throwing away expensive medicine that didn't work out, and keeping a vigilant eye that their spouses did not choke as they tried to swallow their noon handful of pills. Despite their best efforts, sufferers commonly forgot to take their medicines or took them incorrectly. Of course, the return of symptoms served as a reminder, but for many people this reminder came too late. They would take their dose and then wait until their function returned, resentful at having to take the medicine, chastised and irritated by the constant reminders. Caregivers' efforts to minimize their partners' medication use were well intentioned, but sufferers felt they knew best about when and how often to take their pills. Some sufferers, recognizing that the longevity of their good response from carbidopa-levodopa use was limited, took higher doses anyway, believing that they would rather have a few good days than many mediocre ones.

Keeping House

Caregivers often begin their new roles by taking responsibility for health-related chores, finances, and appointments. Over time they find that they are doing a larger and larger share of the household chores, and this shift in the division of labor can be a source of contention between spouses. An eighty-year-old care-giver described these challenges to me: "The challenge has been assuming responsibility for almost all household questions, including financial, for check-ing with doctors, keeping appointments and medications straight. The only reward I see is the slight satisfaction of seeing that one can manage it, at least for the time being. Another challenge is in developing the patience necessary to accommodate to the slowness of movement and of thought in the sufferer, and to the none-too-rare confusion and occasional irritability. I have less time for my own pursuits."

Female caregivers reported that being responsible for everything was very stressful. Their usual duties of laundry, meal preparation, and cleaning are first compounded by the personal care they provide to their spouse. When women have to take on the more physically demanding tasks of yard work, their bodies are doubly taxed and their husbands resentful. Female caregivers acknowledged that their husbands might feel emasculated by seeing their wives mow the lawn, but wives feared the consequences of allowing their spouses to continue mow-ing. On several occasions wives tried to enlist my help in making a case against their husband performing yard work. Although I resisted putting myself in the midst of a marital spat, it was relatively unavoidable. At times I allied with the wives, arguing that mowing the lawn was "risky." Yet I felt badly for husbands and hated to contribute to their already substantial fears.

Male caregivers gained new respect for the nuances of running a house-hold, and men like this seventy-five-year-old caregiver confided to me that they were mystified by the complexity of helping their wives to put on a bra or fix their hair: "I do things for her that I didn't before. I help her get dressed some days, cook, clean, wash clothes, make up her medications, make sure she takes it when she should, decide when she needs to see her doctor and which one. Do all the shopping. Do all of the driving and my work in the yard and care of our home and business."

Several male caregivers approached me for advice on how to help keep up their wives' appearances. They received with great appreciation and slight embarrassment suggestions to switch from back-fastened to pull-on sports bras or from full-length hose to ankle or knee-high stockings and to rely upon weekly hair settings at the local beauty shop. For some men, despite my outsider status,

I was a more socially acceptable source of information than their adult daughters, for whom they strove to maintain every indication of being able to handle caregiving duties.

Part of women's self-worth was wrapped up in their dust-free living rooms, their neatly pressed clothing, and the meals they prepared. Watching their husbands try to cook or clean was tortuous for some female sufferers. Men didn't know how to dust, to properly wash clothes, or to iron. I could imagine the women wincing as their husbands clattered about in the kitchen, making a mess, putting things away in the wrong place, and attempting to cook. Female PD sufferers experience these role shifts as affronts to their femininity.

On the surface, women seemed to find the new demands of caregiving more burdensome than men did. I think there are several reasons for this. First, men were more emotionally reserved and less reflective in their comments to me. Second, women did not always adjust their standards, as male caregivers tended to. For example, when male caregivers took over the kitchen duties, meals became simpler and couples frequented restaurants. Entertaining was unlikely. Men felt that they could provide for their household with frozen dinners. By contrast, women caregivers continued to try to maintain their lifelong standards for cooking and cleaning. This is not to say that women were more inflexible—women did simplify meals and hire housekeepers—but their dignity was expressed in part through these activities. Another factor that may explain the gendered difference I observed in articulating caregiver distress is that when women decided to take over some of their husbands' duties, such as the finances or the auto upkeep, they were frequently devastated by the depth of disorder they discovered. Bills had not been paid for months, records had been misfiled or lost, and mail turned up unopened in an unusual location. Women may have had more catching up to do.

Caregivers working to keep a house a home were at times overwhelmed by the number of their responsibilities. They disliked having to make household decisions alone. Some women quit their jobs to care for their husbands full-time; they missed their work life for its intellectual stimulation, the variety of tasks, and the social interactions work provided. As PD progressed, caregivers begin to dislike leaving their spouse at home alone. Not only can caregivers resent having to take their partners with them, but also they cannot avoid taking them along. Caregivers cannot always maintain the home, and families relocate in anticipation of sufferers' greater dependence and limitations.

Social Life

The people that I met through this study possess myriad talents, interests, travel plans, aspirations, and volunteer positions. I had the pleasure of spending time with people who enjoyed life in whatever capacity they could. Participants valued their leisure time and took part in a variety of hobbies, including woodworking, knitting, quilting, word puzzles, board games, card games and clubs, individual exercise, facilitating a PD support group, scrapbooking and genealogy, philately, gardening, bird watching, reading, writing poetry or memoirs, and watching television or going to movies. They were also busy in a variety of social outlets, including their faith communities (volunteering on boards, leading religious education, or participating in Christian Women's Club or other faith-based groups); and local, regional, or national social organizations such as the Lions Club, Rotary Club, Kiwanis, Optimists Club, PEO, or Red Hats Society. They volunteered—assisting sufferers at the VHA or other hospitals; serving at local parks; participating in political advocacy or advisory groups such as city government or the AARP; and working for public television or at the public library. They spent unstructured time with family or friends, babysat, chatted over coffee in town, and enjoyed recreational travel.

Retirement is often envisioned as a time when one can enjoy life and pass one's days in leisure activities, travel, and enjoying the company of family and friends. The participants in my study had planned to participate in these diverse activities indefinitely, yet PD invariably caused all of them to reduce the number and/or the intensity of involvement. Lillie, sixty-two, described the changes in her caregiving role:

> I've always been the sickly one, with him looking after me. He did lawn and outside work, changing light bulbs, repairs. I am more patient with him. We make decisions together. Now, I'm pretty much responsible for everything. I feel as though I have the role of the mother. He is pretty dependent on me for everything. . . . I have to take his needs into consideration. Previously, I could come and go as I pleased. I can no longer visit my friends for a day, as I try not to leave him for more than two hours at a time. That appears to be changing to shorter time periods as his worsening seems to be progressing. Special challenges [for me are] having to slow down (as in helping him walk) and be much more patient! Not being able to travel any more. I must do all of the driving now, which he mostly did in the past. Our life revolves around his illness.

Caregivers' and sufferers' social engagement diminishes as their ability or willingness to leave the house decreases, as I have mentioned, and as this comment from a seventy-four-year-old caregiver indicates: "He is the same person, yet seems distant. He does not have much interest in things. [He] is slower doing things and he has to be constantly reminded to do things. We used to travel a lot, but he never suggests it anymore. I do most of the driving at the present time. He never suggests doing things. If I didn't say we were doing things, we would sit home all of the time. I have to energize him to do things on his own, without me."

Sufferers I spoke with withdrew because they could no longer keep up with the pace of activities (mentally or physically), they were embarrassed by their symptoms, they received fewer invitations, or they were hindered by their physical impairments (e.g., they can no longer swing that golf club). Sadly, as sufferers' impairments limited their scope of ability and their need for social outlets increased, their social worlds grew smaller.

PD sufferers' social withdrawal puts pressure on caregivers (Murray and Harrison 2004). Caregivers told me they withdrew from social life when they no longer wanted to leave their spouse alone or they no longer had the time to participate. They attended social events solo, but this was less common than simply forgoing their personal interests. Caregivers missed having time for themselves and for enjoying their friendships. They withdrew from social circles, and their social circles withdrew from them. This process did not go unremarked. It angered caregivers and depressed sufferers.

Some caregivers valiantly tried to persuade their spouse to leave the house. Couples went out for drives, dined in restaurants, and went on errands together. The more sufferers withdrew into themselves, the harder their caregivers pushed. Some caregivers interpreted this social aversion as laziness or apathy, and grieved that their partners no longer shared their interests and desires. Wives were embarrassed to attend social functions alone, but they grew tired of having to schedule their social life around pill time, on times, and naps. Sufferers sometimes gave in and accompanied their partners on errands or social outings; nevertheless, the more advanced the case, the more often they preferred to stay home. For as many people who resented others determining their social opportunities, there were an equal number who would rather avoid the questioning glances, embarrassing situations, and exhaustion that accompanied outings and social events.

In Sickness and in Health

Most of the couples I met through this project have been married for forty or more years. Some of them had known each other as children, others had met during or just after World War II, and a few had courted at college. They had shared lean economic times, raised and mourned children, traveled internationally, farmed one hundred or one thousand acres, and made a commitment to grow old together. Over the years, like married couples across the country, some grew more intimate and others drifted apart, held together by an invisible legal thread. As more than one person joked, "Growing old is hell," and the hell of aging stressed already weakening ties. PD's intrusions tested some marriages and reinforced others.

Caregivers sadly reported how difficult it was for them to witness their partner suffering. PD made caregivers feel powerless and ineffectual. As sufferers came to rely upon their spouses, caregivers at times recounted such dependence proudly: "I do feel blue when I realize what my wonderful husband is going through and do worry about his remaining years and what may happen to him," said a seventy-nine-year-old caregiver. "I do not let him know this and always try to be cheerful, but it doesn't always work." And a seventy-six-year-old caregiver told me, "I have grown closer to my wife. We appreciate each other more with each passing year. We believe in the promises of 'for better or for worse' and 'in sickness and in health.' I'm happy that I can still do things for her even though *I* am slowing down."

At other times caregivers chafed under the disorder's unremitting demands: "I find great tact is needed in dealing with his disabilities," said one caregiver, eighty-eight. "It's necessary to smooth things over and, to some extent, keep up the pretense that he can/will do certain things. It's necessary, though sometimes difficult, not to become too directive. It's probably inevitable that one begins to feel that this is not quite the same person one knew before the illness."

Finally, a sixty-nine-year-old caregiver spoke of feeling parental toward her spouse. "It is difficult, as he is becoming more limited all of the time. I find the shuffling and movements annoying, yet I have empathy for him and his problems. I feel it has become or is becoming more of a parent-child relationship. . . . We don't spend as much time just talking and visiting."

Communication problems were an issue that surfaced often. Caregivers (some with hearing impairments) had difficulty deciphering the soft, mumbled speech of their spouse. PD sufferers grew tired of being reminded to speak up, and their partners grew impatient with the repetitive questioning. Cognitive impairments especially taxed caregivers. Husbands became quiet and withdrawn, speaking only when necessary. Wives became angry and combative, adamantly describing their (hallucinatory) version of reality. Caregivers were accused of infidelity and worse. They feared leaving their spouse alone at home, and they missed having someone that they could talk to. Cognitive problems and communication issues were the ones most frequently discussed by caregivers, and changes in couples' intimate relations were broached by a few.

In light of the myriad, individualized affronts of PD on the body, I wondered whether sexual expression was a relevant concern. The literature on sex in PD is extraordinarily thin and focuses on the male sexual experience (Fernandez et al., 2001; Fleming, Tolson, and Schartau 2004; Schreurs, De Ridder, and Bensing 2000). Anorgasmia and impotence are common among PD sufferers (Starkstein and Merello 2002). The questionnaire data that I collected reflects this finding. Thirty-nine percent of PD sufferers and almost half of caregivers reported often having "unsatisfying sexual relations," and about 10 percent of both groups took the time to write in that the question was no longer applicable to their lives.

In the end, I broadened my scope to ask interviewees to describe how PD had affected their relationship with their spouse, allowing participants the flexibility of interpretation. A majority of interviewees chose to answer this question as one of communication and role transition; few discussed their sexuality. One man explained that he was surprised that he could still have a satisfying sexual relationship at his age. Another told me that his antidepressants rendered him impotent and that there was nothing to be done. Two women discussed their sexual health with me. One reported that she had started to lose her sexual response due to muscle stiffness and nervousness. She sought her gynecologist's help and that advice helped her to regain sexual confidence, function, and pleasure. The other woman brought up her intimate life in a discussion of medications. Her neurologist had prescribed a new medication and, when she read through the insert and saw that it could cause sexual dysfunction, she declined to take it. Having had to compromise so much of her independence by allowing her husband to adopt some of what had historically been her household and familial responsibilities, she felt that enough was enough; she was unwilling to risk this further loss in their marital relationship.

Caregivers also provided limited information regarding intimacy in their questionnaire responses. A few caregivers felt that PD had brought them to a deeper level of intimacy with their partner. As one woman explained, "I presume it is because we need each other so much." Caregivers reported that their spouse napped all the time or that they no longer had spontaneous conversations. Sufferers' sleep disturbances, such as frequent night wakings, talking in their sleep, vivid nightmares, or restless legs syndrome, forced some couples to sleep in twin beds. Besides being tired, sometimes revulsed, and lonely for conversation, caregivers found that their role transition made it difficult to find a path to sexual intimacy. Comments such as, "It's more of a parent-child relationship now," and "Sometimes I feel more 'motherly' than 'wifely,'" characterize these changes in their relationships.

Embodiment and Caregiving

The transition to the caregiving role was rarely a complete one. Caregivers' sense of relationship to their partner was connected to the unpredictability of the disease course. Sufferers' needs and impairments changed daily and hourly. Caregivers struggled to predict their husbands' or wives' needs so that their spouses wouldn't be reduced to asking. Sufferers argued that they would rather do for themselves and that they would ask for help if they needed it. Caregivers were faulted by their spouses for providing help too quickly or for waiting too long. Predicting sufferer need on a day-by-day basis was at times overshadowed by the desire of caregivers to know what their lives would be like in five to ten years. Caregivers mourned the loss of their wives' or husbands' confidence and found the signs of progression depressing—"You feel like you are losing them." With deep sadness and many reservations, couples made plans to relocate, wrote living wills, and tried to predict who they would be in the context of pro-gression.

The presence of PD in their lives does not shape caregivers' embodiment of aging in the same ways that it does sufferers'; PD caregiving nonetheless alters caregivers' sense of self and is experienced as a condition or constraint upon their lives. Caregivers enjoyed having more time to spend with their spouse one-on-one. The retirement plans that had been downgraded or abandoned in lieu of running errands or scheduling doctor's appointments provided caregivers with unanticipated and greatly valued time with their partner. Caregiving is frequently discussed in terms of strain and gain, but it is not the specific activities that cause caregiver overload. Instead, it is the meaning that people associate with specific activities or situations that contributes to positive or negative appraisal of the caregiving role (Noonan and Tennstedt 1997). Caregivers in this study felt over-worked, fatigued, and overwhelmed, and these feelings contributed to a larger sense of aging more rapidly than they had expected. Their partner's increasing needs had sped up what they had anticipated would be a gradual progression to a simpler social calendar and more frequent doctor's visits.

However, their transition to the caregiving role provided unexpected satis-factions that counterbalance this acceleration. Caregivers explained that they gained a more profound sense of self by taking care of another person. Their role gave them a bigger purpose in life; they were reaching out beyond them-selves to help their spouse. This role gave them great satisfaction, knowing that they could accomplish a position that was so important, so taxing, and so valu-able to their loved one. Caregivers were proud of their abilities to manage their household and the needs of their husbands or wives. Despite feeling that they were also "old before their time," caregivers were assisting their partners in aging gracefully. Caregiving was a role that helped to sustain them through their periods of anticipatory grief and the management of chronic sorrow.

9

Conclusion

Aging, Embodiment, and Conditions

Introduction: Have You Come Up with a Cure Yet?

In the lazy postlunch hour the support group members and I found seats around the conference table. Everett brought the meeting to order and slowly everyone drew their private conversations to a close and gave him their attention. Everett suggested that we go around the table and each say a few words about how we were doing.

EVERETT: I have been doing pretty well this past month. I can't sleep at night, but that is nothing new. I wake up four or five times a night—I bet I get about five hours of sleep a night. My golf swing isn't what it used to be. I imagine that this will be the last season for that. I am walking, though, almost every day. No change to my medications lately. How about you, Edgar?

EDGAR: Me? Oh, I am doing all right. I was in the hospital for a few days this past month, on account of my lung problems. I have COPD, you know. That gives me more trouble than the PD does. The main problem I have is the tremor. Drives me crazy. But, it's really my lungs that are the worst. I can handle the tremor, but I don't like having to [take my COPD medication] too much.

It was Hazel's turn. Hazel had been losing weight and looked to be down to about a hundred pounds. She was thin and weak. With her eyes closed and her head bobbing, she struggled to speak. She raised her hands, ropy and frail birds fluttering about her face. Her husband spoke for her: "She's got tremor real bad, too. Nothing they can do for it anymore. She has her good days, but the tremor just shakes the weight right off of her. Hazel's now taking more than twenty pills a day, between her heart and her PD and her osteoporosis. It's a wonder she can eat with all of them."

Another woman explained that she had been having recurrent headaches and called her doctor for advice. He had lowered her dose of carbidopa-levodopa and added venlaxafine HCL. She elaborated: "I am also taking mirtaza-pine for sleep. My tremor has been getting worse and I have been seeing things. I keep seeing other people in the room, and I know they aren't there. The other day I kept imagining that my husband was out working. I wish he'd bring home some money! [laughs] The psychiatrist said that I need to change my medica-tions again. I am going back in a few weeks, but I guess they want to get one more experiment in before then."

The man seated to her right gripped the table tightly with both hands and looked around the room. His tremor was going full force today—hands, arms, and head shaking. His glasses kept sliding down his nose, and he looked pretty banged up. He stammered with effort, "I've been all right. I took a bad spill the other week, but I am doing ok."

His wife added, Yes, you did, didn't you? I was asleep and the next thing I knew I had gotten a phone call from the church. [My husband] had gotten up out of bed and gone off to the church. It wasn't the church that we attend, but someone who was outside in the parking lot there knew who he was and saw him trip and fall over the curb. They called me right away to come get him." She chuckled. "You were still in your pajamas, weren't you?"

It was my turn to share. Wallace asked me, "Have you found a cure yet?" I blushed and countered, "Well, I know of one way to get over it, but I bet no one's in a rush to go that route!" We all shared a bit of a laugh over that. I joked because I was not sure how to respond. To respond directly would be to draw into the discussion a sense of gravity that would noticeably change the tenor of the day's meeting. I went on to assure everyone that I was indeed learning a great deal and to remind them that I wasn't looking for some "right answer" but that I was wanting to observe, discuss, and see firsthand what it was like to live with PD. The conversation moved on to other topics, but a sense of uneasiness regarding my responsibility remained with me.

I had been welcomed into people's homes, been witness to indignities, shared tears, and been privy to the intimate details of their failing and uncon-trollable bodies. When I brought my fieldwork to a close, the initial reserve with which I had been treated had largely dissipated. In drawing me into the embrace of their lives, people recognized my commitment to understanding their expe-riences. This commitment and responsibility is often talked about in anthropol-ogy in terms of representation, of providing a space for situated voices to speak to power. For those of us who work with what are often termed "special" or "vul-nerable" populations, the commitment and responsibility deepens. Despite anthropology's self-consciousness about a disciplinary preoccupation with the exotic other, the field continues to privilege study of the underdog, the disen-franchised, and the culturally distant. Anthropologists working with older adults, and especially those living with a stigmatizing disorder such as PD, are at times hyperaware of our motivations for research and the ethical implications of how we communicate our findings. Simply put, from my first day of fieldwork to today, I have been careful to represent PD sufferers as neither heroes nor tragic victims.

Self-representation has also figured prominently in my concern to produce a text that is both scholarly and accessible, both humanly compelling and theoretically grounded. Yet I have to admit to having written the book with a slight glance over my shoulder, with a self-consciousness regarding my own age and a recognition of the relatively low status afforded "domestic research" within anthropology. I have had many conversations with other anthropologists who study populations "at home," bemoaning the biases we as anthropologists have against doing ethnography among our own people, railing against the idea that North Americanists are less theoretically sophisticated, too politically motivated, too close to their research community to be reasonably objective, or that we choose to do research in the United States because of convenience or due to our inability to hack it overseas in "real" field sites. Slightly less often have I been drawn into discussions of the new acceptance of anthropology at home, citing the rich history of prominent scholars who chose to work in North America and did so with sophistication and aplomb. More than these undercurrents in the field, however, is my own observation that is has been less my choice of field site that gives colleagues pause (though many laugh at the idea of Iowa having culture) than my choice of study population. As I joke with a colleague who works with orphaned street children: "Why would you want to expose yourself to that? How depressing." The image of older adults as boring, depressing, and inevitably declining until death, as Myerhoff (1978) noted more than thirty years ago now, pushes many U.S. anthropologists away from work with this interesting, lively, and important population. Yet my colleagues (outside geroanthropology) were not the only ones to wonder why I chose to do research among this vulnerable group—PD sufferers themselves frequently joked that I was too young to be spending my afternoons listening to their stories and watching their struggles.

I strive to be critical of how my own life course trajectory has structured what I am able to see and hear in the field, but I also take care to practice an "economy of disclosure" (Leibing and McLean 2007). That is, throughout the book I've aimed to be a visible actor whose social and somatic location shapes both my inquiry and what I am able to see and hear in response. As the number of months since my last support group meeting increases, so do the number of deaths and the burden of disability sustained by individual sufferers. At the outset of fieldwork I knew that I would see terrible things—people in unremitting pain, depression, grief, stigma, and conflict—and that there would be little that I could do to relieve this suffering. I also knew that death would come and that sometimes it would be welcomed and at other times questioned. What I hadn't counted on was how these experiences would intensify the work of communicating the experiences I was privy to. My informal conversations with other geroanthropologists reveal a shared sense of emotional and personal responsibility for representing and explaining elders' experiences without resorting to exoticizing them to gain disciplinary cachet or interest. These interactions also indicate the lack of academic space for revealing the personal costs of working with disenfranchised aging people. Rather than employ a sense of struggle to describe my own lesser work (those living with PD have the greater occupation), I think it helpful to view fieldwork with the chronically sick or aging not as a burden of responsibility, but as a process of reflecting the human capacity to empathize and a desire to understand, to create meaning.

As many tears as I have shed alone in my hotel room after conducting an interview or holding the hand of a caregiver across the kitchen table, there have been as many moments of brightness and enjoyment. PD is not a life sentence of encroaching disability and suffering until death, but it is not an easy condition with which to live. The challenge for me has been to communicate a sense of being in the sufferer's body without having dwelled in a PD-stricken form. A hoarse voice raised in despair or jest; a drawn face masking an inner world of feeling; a soft hand grasping the back of a chair to steady the standing body; and eyes scanning the ceiling for those important links which string words into language—these are the conduits of communication.

Throughout the book I've aimed to integrate anthropological, clinical, and other academic literature with the ethnographic view. This integration arises from the recognition that PD sufferers themselves are not divorced or isolated from these circulating discourses about their condition. It also serves as a reminder that embodiment occurs in a cultural space constructed by competing claims to authority and truth. The challenge of writing in this way has been to bring together disparate perspectives on equal footing, to slip between biomedical jargon, sufferer narratives, and anthropological theory, at once respecting their claims and situating them as variants on a theme. An anthropology of aging is not necessarily an anthropology of the body, but in the case of PD, the embodiment of aging is forever enacted through a somatic being in the world and the expectation of an unpredictable senescence.

Between Wellness and Sickness, Illness and Disease: PD and Other Conditions

A condition is a state of being which lies between complete health and descent into sickness, but also between the two poles of sickness experience—disease and illness. It marks a special category of experience, akin to but different from an interminable sick role. Having a condition means that one never fully identities with the sick role but is rarely without the consciousness of having to live within the parameters set by one's disorder. Living with a condition also reflects the changing relationship between illness and disease in U.S. biomedicine. Biomedical authority retains its legitimacy and power, yet the sick are forging paths toward greater access to biomedical scholarship, to participate in clinical trial development, to advocate for research funding for their own disease, and to gain a stronger foothold in medical decision-making encounters.

A condition is a qualifier of embodiment, an ever-present variable negotiated over the remainder of the life course. It speaks to and hints at limitation, but does not guarantee it. Accordingly, sufferers find ways to reshape their lives and desires around the demands conditions set, but they do so in a nuanced context with recognized temporal, interpersonal, and somatic variables. Chronic illness sufferers arrive at the diagnostic moment with an illness perspective; over time, as they are encouraged to take an active role in the ongoing management of their sickness, they begin to adopt medical terminology and to interpret their somatic bodies in light of biomedical theory. The temporal nature of chronic disorders transforms an illness into a condition. Conditions present an uncertain prognosis and an often-indeterminate etiology, warrant lifelong medical management, and are incurable.

The uncertainty that conditions promise is accompanied by a qualifier to one's sense of identity. Conditions do not necessarily compel biographical disruption, but they do often foment a life course transition. As sufferers' conditions vary in their intrusiveness, so does the ability of sufferers to retain their familiar metric for assessing their current abilities (see Ohman and Lundman 2003). As much as a condition is something unique about afflicted persons, a quality of their bodies with which they contend, it is very often something which sufferers seek to downplay, control, manage, or hide. These processes are driven not so much by inner shame at being unable to continue to use one's personal history to define one's current identity, as by societal pressures to retain that historical narrative. Sufferers may use these processes of obfuscation to avoid situations where other people's definitions for who they should be and of what their proper behavior should consist come to determine their social worlds.

In chapter 1 I explained my choice of the word "sufferer" to refer to elders living with PD. At first I hesitated to adopt this term because of its negative connotation and because very few Iowan elders with PD would openly consider themselves to be "suffering." Yet the term remains a good fit ideologically, for it reminds us that the suffering from conditions such as PD is not solely the product of somatic limitation or inadequate coping. Suffering in conditions is a social process. Suffering is a relational process. Physicians and other social actors view a PD sufferer's body from their own standard of able-bodiedness or beauty and make assumptions about which symptoms are the source of suffering for that other person. These assumptions, if divorced from a biographical narrative that can lay meaning onto somatic disorder, serve to intensify the suffering experience.

PD is not the sole disorder that we can consider a condition. Its symptoms possess similarities to the experience of other chronic diseases, introduced in chapter 1 but worth revisiting here. Rheumatoid arthritis, a disfiguring and painful disorder, is also experienced not as an illness identity but sometimes as an affliction that one adjusts to (Stamm et al. 2008). MS is a disease that shares PD's unpredictable course, enervation, and mobility impairments. MS sufferers derive a sense of impairment from context, from the disabling environments in which they operate (Reynolds and Prior 2003). MS sufferers may not identify as sick, nor would they consider themselves truly well (Ingadottir and Halldorsdottir 2008), but they may also be reticent to identify as "someone who has MS," choosing to consider MS as another aspect of their identity and experience that creates a qualifier of their embodiment (Monks 1995). Similarly, diabetes sufferers may resist adopting the label "diabetic" and instead choose to consider diabetes part of their identity or one of a number of factors they contend with in daily life (Ingadottir and Halldorsdottir 2008).

Rather than invent a new term to mark my place in the disciplinary jargon, examining and discarding existing tools and theories as outmoded or limited, I intend my discussion of condition to build upon our understanding of illness narratives and explanatory models, and I structured the ethnographic chapters accordingly. The diagnostic process, embarked upon with the promise of resolution and treatment, emerges as the initiating moment of embodiment rather than the endpoint. Once diagnosed with PD, sufferers come to understand that their life with this disease fails to fit into a preestablished model for symptoms and progression. Instead, PD is an individual disease and operates as a set of related somatic and cognitive conditions which act as qualifiers on elders' aging process. Efforts to define PD, pathologically or functionally, bring into play competing claims to authority. Clinicians' opinions differ as to which symptoms are definitive—narrower definitions lower the number of PD sufferers, while broader guidelines may introduce too many sufferers of atypical PD. PD sufferers incorporate biomedical information into their own models for understanding the disorder. Thus, PD becomes a condition defined by the most life-altering intrusiveness it presents. Sufferers' explanations of what PD is reflect the narrowing gap between lay and expert knowledge. People incorporate medical knowledge, although not in a scientifically rigorous way, into their autobiographical narrative, electing to highlight certain aspects of culpability and downplay others.

The challenge of the management of PD symptoms is that the heterogeneity of cases is matched by an equally complex pharmacopoeia. That the medications failed to restore normal function, that they possess their own progression of decreasing efficacy, and that they may work well one day and seem ineffective the next—all emphasize the conditional nature of sufferers' control over their bodies. Several sufferers, continuing to take medications that they felt had no effect on their symptoms, reflect the power of biomedical authority to control hope and compliance, even in the context of inadequate relief. Finally, the variability of progression and disease course subtly demonstrate the conditional nature of life with PD. PD is a condition unique to the individual and one that promises decline. Sufferers know enough to recognize that greater accommodations will likely have to be made, but they can't see in what order symptoms will present, or how quickly they may slide into the space where the body can no longer respond to the heart's desire.

Narrative, Embodiment, and Aging

As a condition, the embodiment of PD differs according to individual sufferers' social location. The age of older adults with PD influences the ways in which they regard the limitations PD presents. Sufferers' efforts to make sense of their experiences through the idioms of age and PD reveal that age continues to be defined as a process of decline, expressed primarily through the somatic body. The adage "You are only as old as you feel" rings true, but it is clear that how we feel remains an intersection of the individual, culture, and somatic. These intersections are evident when examining the economic and social constraints of PD sufferers, but they are more readily understood via sufferers' illness narratives, an autobiographical life course perspective.

Anthropologists have always been interested in stories, although the seriousness with which we attend to them has varied. Feminist ethnography (e.g., Behar and Gordon 1996; Wolf 1992) and the "narrative turn" in anthropology inspired a reconsideration of the function and meaning of the stories that people share. Mattingly (1998) provides an excellent discussion of the strengths and quandaries of the narrative turn in anthropology. According to her, narratives can be read in three ways—as straightforward accounts of past events, as cultural scripts that teach proper behavior and beliefs from particular cultural and historical locations, or as performances with some deeper function for the performer and the audience. And, as Wolf's (1992) work has cleverly demonstrated, each reading tells only a partial tale. The fragmented nature of these texts is due to the disconnect between narrative and experience. As Mattingly argues, narrative does not reflect experience, but rather narratives are intertextual. "What is needed is a *theory of emergent meaning* that does the following: (a) recognizes the place of cultural scripts but also the importance of immediate contexts; (b) acknowledges the powerful role of discourse in shaping meaning, but also attends to non-linguistic action; (c) accounts not only for the public meanings shared by a cultural group but offers a means for interpreting private meanings, the 'inner landscape' of an individual's motives, desires, beliefs, emotions" (1998, 44; emphasis added).

What Mattingly has called a theory of emergent meaning has been employed in the recent (re)discovery of the body and embodiment. Csordas, a major contributor to this stimulating direction, positions embodiment as a paradigm for cultural anthropology: "This approach to embodiment begins from the methodological postulate that the body is not an object to be studied in relation to culture, but is to be considered as the subject of culture, or in other words as the existential ground of culture" (1990, 5). As cultural creations and creators, we both have bodies and are bodies, and our experience of the body is integrally connected to our notions of identity and self (Hockey and James 2003). Embodiment is an epistemological tool for integrating the somatic, social, spiritual, gendered, aging, and other bodies. It occurs in the space between the body and culture and is communicated via the ways in which people interpret and create meaning from particular social locations.

The embodiment of age is culturally constructed and autobiographically unique. Becker's (1997) work on biographical disruption illustrates how somatic phenomena affect the self (see also Bury 1982). The loss of self is a "disrupted embodiment"—in the context of chronic or disabling illness, sufferers are no longer the persons they once were (Murray and Harrison 2004). But embodiment is not hegemonic, and people can resist the dominant form of embodiment by choosing to experience their bodies in a different way (Charlton and Barrow 2002). The embodiment of disease as a condition supports the multifactoral nature of somatic experience. As Charmaz has noted (1983, 1991), the somatic is one piece of the suffering produced in sickness, and the chronically ill may be as limited by social mores as they are by their unique impairments. The construction of identity is an interactional and lifelong process (Charmaz 1991; see also Settersten 2003), but while diagnosis may foment a moment of disruption, it is the interactions between individuals, their bodies, their social world, and their autobiographical narratives which come to constitute their condition.

As cultural processes and categories, aging and sickness are related. They both possess temporal frameworks of acceptability, are frequently associated with lower social status, have the potential to foment suffering, and draw the body into the foreground of being. Aging is a cultural process that is stratified by historically contingent social factors, such as gender, race, ethnicity, marital status, economic class, educational attainment, or physical ability. In the United States, social aging seems inextricably linked with appearance and the physical body. Age is ascribed to such signs as gray hair, baldness, wrinkles, slowness, bifocals, the use of assistive devices such as a cane or walker, possession of an accessible parking pass, stooped posture, increased reaction time, or prescription drug use. And despite age-positive advertisements that target aging baby boomers as an antiestablishment generation who will age differently, the proliferation of consumer goods to hide, deny, or forestall outward signs of aging confirms the negative associations of older age with decreased status. Aging is marked not only by chronological age and the body, but also by the use of out-moded clothing, automobiles, or language. Some of these markers are innocu-ous, others are the targets of gentle intergenerational teasing, and a few are the grounds for age-based discrimination. As well as mechanisms for social exclu-sion, markers such as these are means by which elders find shared status as older adults.

When older people begin to take note of their display of such age-related social markers, when they recognize their own aging, the practice of embodi-ment of age changes. No longer are somatic annoyances such as generalized slowness or backache seen as transitory complaints: Oftentimes the somatic becomes enveloped by aging. Older people certainly do seek treatment for their maladies, be they general or specific, and there are chronic and acute sicknesses that arise more frequently in later life. And yet the story that I expected to find—that older people interpret early, generalized PD symptoms as normal aging—was not the universal narrative diagnosed PD sufferers shared with me. Instead, PD illness narratives spoke to a more complex relationship with social aging. A PD diagnosis does not resolve the question, Is this a sign of old age or a sign of disease?—it merely changes its dynamic. Sufferers accept that PD is not old age, but they continue to ask their bodies, "Is this old age or PD?" in order to identify the proper performance of age and disease status. After diagnosis, the embodi-ment of aging becomes expressed through the somatic body.

By virtue of their diagnosis, PD sufferers come to measure their aging by a somatic metric. Their explanatory models, as presented in chapters 3 through 7, reveal that they distinguish PD from aging, but that they view both processes as promising inevitable decline. Their narratives speak to the importance of sepa-rating normal aging from disease because this separation informs them how to appropriately perform each mode of being in the world. Chronological age emerged as a prominent variable in shaping these performances, as each decade of life was associated with a narrative that emphasized how PD acceler-ates, mediates, or obscures aging.

In the case of PD, the process of determining whether one is sick or simply aging is complicated by varying clinical standards for diagnosis, by the disor-der's typically slow onset, and by the overlap of PD symptoms with signs of nor-mal aging. Neither age at onset nor presenting symptoms was associated with the length of time from onset to diagnosis. The diagnostic moment and doctor-patient communication mark the onset of transformation in sufferers' embodi-ment of aging. Physicians' comments that greater age at onset was positive because life had already been lived expose providers' negative views of later life.

For people in their sixties, the markers of age arrived earlier than expected. Such people commonly remarked on feeling cheated by life and the ways in which they appeared to be older than their years. Their unsmiling faces, slowed movement, and stooped posture were markers of an old age that they were not yet ready to experience. Daily and lifelong medication use, with the prospect of increasing dosages with decreasing efficacy, widened the gap between the age they wanted to perform and the one they were being drawn to perform. When considering their prognosis, PD sufferers in their sixties were daunted by the notion that dependency might arrive sooner than later, and they worried about maintaining private insurance to pay for prescription medication costs, as well as their lack of access to certain kinds of insurance due to their diagnosis. This shaped their embodiment of aging such that PD accelerated the aging process. Their narratives explained that physical impairments are acceptable in later life, but that they themselves were not yet *old*. They define PD and aging similarly but attribute the ultimate causes differently.

For those in the middle-old group, aged seventy to seventy-nine, PD came to mediate the embodiment of aging. The mediating narrative told a story of separation: PD and aging were separate processes, and it was important to these people to distinguish between the two. Mediators described their frustrations with physicians who would refuse or were otherwise unable to tell them whether their symptoms could be attributed to PD or aging. The phrase "a straight answer," used repeatedly, called attention to the stakes of enacting this separation. Among older Iowans, and especially rural-dwelling ones, self-reliance and independence are key markers of integrity and community standing. Being in a position of having to ask for help is fraught with feelings of inadequacy and ingratitude. Some people confided to me that they would rather die than be dependent upon others, be seen as an object of pity. Others explained that to complain about one's maladies is a sign of ingratitude. Thus, being able to determine which somatic changes can be tied to PD gives sufferers a socially acceptable way to voice their human frailties. Asking for help because one has a disease is more acceptable than asking for help simply because one is getting older.

The PD sufferers aged eighty and older shared narratives that viewed aging in a different light. Perhaps because their chronological age placed them closer to death, discussion of aging was strikingly absent. Rather, this group for whom PD obscures aging linked virtually all the social and somatic changes in their lives to their PD status. When they were no longer able to drive, or when they could not maintain their farmhouse and had to move into town, it was because of their PD and not because of their greater age. If a new symptom arose, it was commonly thought of as part of PD progression and not always interrogated as perhaps normal aging or even as a symptom of comorbidity. However, a handful of people in this group resisted the envelopment of aging by their diagnosis. Their narratives told stories of physicians' refusal to consider that new symptoms might be a sign of something other than PD progression.

PD reflects and reproduces the prevailing cultural context that constructs aging as an inevitable decline. When sufferers say that they feel old before their time, they are at once reflecting and reproducing the embodiment of aging as an inexorable decline. The symptoms of PD that overlap with stereotypical markers of older age cause sufferers to wonder if they are getting old or if something is really wrong. At that moment patients' experience of PD is mediating aging—the border between normal and abnormal aging is being determined. The function of PD as an obscurer of aging demonstrates how sufferers' embodiment can be indicative of the ongoing medicalization of aging.

The concept of conditions and the ways in which PD influences the embodiment of aging are part of a scholarly discourse that PD sufferers may access but not fully utilize in their daily endeavors to live with this condition. What I hope they do utilize is the context provided by other sufferers' narratives. Everett once shared the following joke with me about life with PD:

OPPORTUNITIES FOR PD PATIENTS

Cameraman for movies simulating earthquakes

Percussionist for music featuring drum rolls

Tester in a telegraph key factory

Movie extras for scenes where the gunman yells, "Freeze!"

Threading a running sewing machine

Butter churn

His sense of humor, and comments from PD sufferers such as Edna, who explained, "We are aging gracefully, Samantha. Trying. Some days are not as graceful as the others," provide a space for PD sufferers to recognize themselves. In doing so, may their recognition be one of camaraderie and fellowship in a life with shaking hands.

APPENDIX A
INTERVIEW PARTICIPANTS

Allen is eighty years old and has had PD for five years. His PD is akinetic and he is quick to point out his physical and memory-related failings. He has recently undergone gastrointestinal surgery, the results of which cause him greater impairment than his PD. Allen's slowness and imbalance make him feel as if he cannot be relied upon, though his wife is quick to remind him of his abilities and contributions.

Andrew is sixty-four years old and has had PD for more than fifteen years. He has a history of depression and anxiety, but his PD presented with postural instability and discoordination. Andrew feels strongly positive about his medications and physicians, and augments these successes with a daily walking routine. For him, PD is one of those things that happens as you get older and is a burden that he must bear without complaining, for in his estimation it could be far worse.

Anna is seventy-three years old and has had PD for about ten years. Her PD causes severe bradykinesia and postural instability. She explains that she always feels tired and that she cannot keep up with a conversation or a television program. Anna has been feeling sad about her husband's encroachment on the kitchen duties, and they are negotiating the new terrain as her physical impairments begin to preclude her from preparing meals, dressing herself, or cleaning her home.

Anthony is in his midsixties and works full-time at a restaurant. PD has affected his executive function, particularly his ability to place his body in space, and this change has started to interfere with his work. He has difficulty maintain the fast pace required of restaurant work and regrets sharing news of his diagnosis with his employer, whom Anthony now feels looks for reasons to fire him. Anthony must continue to work to be able to pay for his apartment and living expenses. He is widowed and has no financial support from children or other family.

Audrey is a sixty-year-old caregiver to her husband, Glen. Caring for her husband and having to place him in a long-term care facility have tested her faith and taxed her body. She is ten years younger than her partner and has felt that his condition aged her before her time. She visits her husband daily and is slowly regaining her strength after years of sleep deprivation and her own medical problems.

Bonnie is in her early sixties and has had PD for more than ten years. She and her husband continue to operate a medium-sized farm and she works part-time in retail for supplemental income. Bonnie's mother has AD, and Bonnie's own recent memory lapses leave her fearing the worst. She has taken memory aid courses and multivitamins to ward off dementia, but she also recognizes that her PD is progressing. Bonnie waited as long as possible before beginning carbidopa-levodopa therapy, and now must take several PD medications to maintain the delicate balance among motor function, rigidity, and dyskinesia.

Clifford is seventy years old and has had PD for two years. He describes his symptoms as lack of ambition, lost voice, and shaking hands. Clifford lives on the farm where he was raised. He continues to operate several farms with the help of his family and a newly hired farm manager. Clifford is very frustrated by what he sees as his inability to get going and get to work, and he complains that the PD medications have no positive effect.

Clyde is sixty-two years old and still employed full-time. He diagnosed his own PD and has been treating his tremor for about ten years. PD has not slowed Clyde's busy medical practice nor changed his retirement plans. While his tremor and rigidity do affect his dexterity, PD medications seem to be providing him with adequate function.

David is seventy-two years old and has had PD for about five years. His PD has caused generalized body aches and pains, slowness, and loss of dexterity. David finds that distinguishing between PD and older age is not easy and perhaps in the end not that useful an enterprise. He feels that his current condition is a result of working hard and treating his body roughly. While he does suffer from unpredictable emotionality, David tries to focus on his abilities rather than his disabilities.

Edgar is seventy-six years old and has had PD for at least five years. He attributes his PD to his work-related exposure to pesticides and recalls several instances where pesticide exposure made him feel ill and shaky. Now retired, Edgar finds his PD causes a moderate unilateral tremor and soft speech. His PD seems unresponsive to the usual medications, and he wonders if he should continue taking them if they have no outwardly visible benefit.

Edna is seventy-four years old and has had PD for twenty years. Her symptoms have been mild and slow progressing, which allowed Edna to continue her extensive community volunteerism until recently. Her husband has retired, and he has begun taking over some of Edna's household duties. This shift in their relationship has caused some tension. Edna resents having to ask for help but also dislikes it when her husband automatically does something for her. Her husband struggles with trying to predict situations where she will need help but avoiding "butting in" and making her feel helpless.

Eileen is sixty-eight years old and has had PD for more than thirty years. She has had DBS surgery on both sides of her brain but still relies upon medications and suffers from debilitating tremor and postural instability. Her PD causes frequent falls, yet she perseveres in walking independently, believing that acceptance of assistive devices will be a slippery slope toward dependence.

Ethel is sixty years old and has had PD for five years. Her tremor is slight, but her slowness forced her to retire early. She suffers from serious depression, speaks slowly, and can walk only a few yards at a time. Ethel is socially active with women much older than she, which affects her sense of self and future. Her especially doting husband now takes care of all of the household chores and driving.

Eva is eighty-four years old and has lived with PD for about four years. She has a history of depression and has had to take care of her husband and adult child, both of whom died a few years before her PD presented. Eva has considerable balance impairment and falls often. She jokes about setting records for falling and not breaking bones, but she does worry about the frequency and severity of her accidents. She takes a handful of PD medications several times a day and manages her care more or less independently.

Everett is in his eighties and has had PD for about ten years. He struggles with a soft, slurred voice, stooped posture, balance problems, and slowness. Everett has trouble staying awake during the day and staying asleep at night. His medication window is getting smaller by the year, but he has a positive outlook. He has recently self-restricted his driving to a sixty-mile radius of his home and has had to give up golf for fear of falling over. Everett perseveres in walking regularly and stays socially active, dining at restaurants, attending concerts, and serving in several community organizations.

Glenn is seventy-two years old and has had PD for eight years. He can no longer walk or dress himself unassisted and he has limited ability to hold a conversation. He can answer direct simple questions and can speak reflectively about the past. He feels badly that his wife, Audrey, has had to care for him and that she suffers from her decision to move him to a facility.

Gordon is seventy-two years old and has had PD for fifteen years. His PD is akinetic and his main problems are confusion, slowness, and anxiety. He was working full-time when PD presented, and his employers moved him to successively less-demanding positions until he was forced to retire before his sixtieth birthday. Gordon experiences hallucinations daily and rarely speaks. He ventures that his inability to communicate normally is a burden to his wife, who he conceded must be lonely and frustrated.

Grace is eighty-five years old and has had PD for about ten years. She has a mild tremor and balance impairment, but her primary complaint lately has been depression. Grace went through a troublesome period of establishing the balance between mobility and cognition and experienced scary medication-induced hallucinations. She and her husband live in a modest suburban home and on their daily walks she prefers to hold onto her husband instead of a cane.

Harold is eighty-two years old and has had PD for about nine years. He has a moderate tremor in one hand and describes long restless nights. Harold owns several farms but is no longer actively involved in their daily operations. He worries more about dementia and cancer than about the loss of his physical ability and is especially concerned about the well-being of his wife should he become incapacitated by PD.

Harry is seventy-nine years old and has had PD for almost a decade. He lives with his wife, Jennie, in a small two-story suburban home. In addition to giving him the mask, PD has contributed to Harry's stooped posture and slow, shuffling walk. Over the past five years Harry has had to relinquish a number of household responsibilities, such as driving, taking out the trash, and running the snow blower. These losses and other people's assessments of his ability to participate have slowly shrunk his circle of influence. Harry hasn't taken these changes quietly and strives to stay as active as possible.

Hazel is an eighty-three-year-old retired schoolteacher diagnosed with PD ten years ago. Her initial symptom was slowness, for which her family urged her to seek care. Hazel demurred, explaining that she would feel silly going to the doctor just because she was slow. Eventually she agreed and learned that she had PD. Since that time she has lost a great deal of weight, has become unsteady on her feet, trembles, and loses her balance. Hazel lived with her husband of more than fifty years in a small apartment; they recently relocated to an assisted-living facility.

Helen is sixty-five years old and has had PD for more than ten years. Her PD began with a mild tremor, which has progressed to a moderate tremor, postural instability, and restless legs. She is lively and outgoing, an avid reader, and lives by herself in a well-appointed town house. Helen is frustrated by her slowness and is increasingly angered by the disconnect between her intention and her movement.

Henry is eighty-two years old and has had PD for more than fifteen years. He is plagued by a moderate and persistent tremor that interferes with writing, eating, dressing, and reading. Henry suffers from depression, and this retired educator is grieved by his inability to read, write, or communicate effectively. He dislikes dining out or making social calls, preferring the solitude of his home. His balance problems and hallucinations have become a source of stress in his marriage. His wife has recently started using respite services and reports that this is an important outlet for her.

Irene is in her early seventies and caregiver to Gordon. She is a petite woman, and it is hard to imagine her helping Gordon up from a fall or trying to deter him from the immediacy of his "waking dreams." Irene performs all the household responsibilities and has begun to leave Gorden in adult day care in order to have some time to herself and to run errands on her own like shopping or going to the post office.

Jack is seventy-two years old and has had PD for a few years. He woke up one morning to find his arm shaking and began a two-year search for an answer. He was initially diagnosed with AD; only recently was the diagnosis changed to PD. He continues to work part-time on construction projects and is physically active. Jack has trouble staying focused and cries easily. His PD has more cognitive than physical involvement, which sets him apart from other people at the support group and leads him to wonder about the nature of PD. He takes the usual PD medications to control his tremor, as well as antipsychotics to ameliorate his cognitive changes.

Jeanne is sixty-seven years old. She was diagnosed with PD in her early sixties, a capstone to a tremendously stressful year. She strives to keep her disease status private, even as she recognizes that others can increasingly see her tremor and instability. Jeanne has a close-knit family who has closed ranks to support her—a move that she both appreciates and feels limited by. She is widowed, lives alone, and maintains a busy social calendar with friends, grandchildren, church, and her pets.

Jennie is a wife and caregiver to Harry. She is in her early seventies and is outraged by the cost of her and Harry's medications. She hauled out their shoebox-sized baskets of prescriptions, explained how much each cost, and shared with me her concern that their private insurance would drop the prescription drug benefit when Medicare D took effect. She provides transportation and some organizational support to Harry. She continues to perform a majority of the housekeeping duties despite her own chronic conditions, and the couple hires help for some of the outside tasks that Harry is no longer able to do.

Joe is sixty-four years old and has had PD for about ten years. Joe has moderate to severe dementia and is troubled by his memory loss. He walks with assistance and difficulty and falls often. He has difficulty initiating conversation and eats and speaks slowly.

June is eighty-four and has had PD for four years. Her PD seems well controlled, though she has had a tremendously difficult time with medication side effects. At times her medications have caused disturbing hallucinations so realistic that she has called the sheriff to investigate. She lives alone, venturing out infrequently to the grocery store, to play cards with friends, or to the support group.

Kathryn is a caregiver of and married to Leroy. She is in her midsixties and has been retired for about five years. Kathryn works hard to protect Leroy both from the consequences of his overestimating his abilities and from a larger society that over time ostracizes slow-moving people.

Laura was recently widowed when Peter, her husband of more than fifty years, died. She had complete responsibility for all the housekeeping, financial, transportation, and social arrangements in their lives. Peter was able to dress and bathe himself, but Laura assisted with tasks that require manual dexterity, such as zipping Peter's pants or pouring his coffee. Her own age, health issues, and small stature made caring for Peter a considerable risk and she sadly moved him to a nursing home.

Lawrence is eighty-one years old and has had PD for at least seven years. His PD has slowed him down, but the medications keep his tremor and postural hypotension well managed. Lately he says that he feels a sort of uneasiness around the time that he is due to take his next dose of medicine, but overall he feels good and is pleased with his life. Lawrence spends his days watching television, reading, and puttering in the back yard. He no longer drives and consequently doesn't get to fish much anymore. He lives with his wife of sixty-one years in an affluent suburban neighborhood.

Leroy is sixty-nine years old and had had PD for seven years. He has the typical PD posture and gait and is becoming increasingly frail and thin. Leroy is frustrated by an ever-shortening medication window and has had some embarrassing incidents as a result of the on/off effect. The unpredictability of his motor function leads him to turn down social invitations and make fewer travel plans. These changes have saddened him and have tightened the range of social activities for his wife as well.

Lillian is seventy-two years old and has never been married. She had a career in sales and as a retiree stays busy with a number of volunteer positions around town. She was diagnosed about a year before we met and had symptoms of PD for about a year and a half prior to that. Her PD is characterized by slowness, mild unilateral tremor, and drowsiness. Lillian has never been on PD medications but is considering relocating to more accessible housing in anticipation of greater physical impairments.

Liza is seventy-seven years old and has lived with PD for twenty-five years. She suffers from postural instability, depression, and fatigue. Liza cannot walk any distance, does not drive, and can no longer prepare family meals or orchestrate holiday events. She has never seen a neurologist for her care, and though she requires a great deal of assistance with things from dressing to shopping, her family does not employ any outside help. Liza admits to being depressed and worries about what may happen to her should her husband's health fail.

Lorraine is married to Richard and is semiretired. Her nursing background has been a tremendous help to Richard's treatment, and she serves as his advocate. They have been married more than forty years, but she is growing tired of the sleepless nights and Richard's insistence that other people are in their home. She cannot leave him alone in the house for very long anymore.

Lucille is in her early seventies and has had PD for about five years. Her first symptom was a hand tremor when she was doing things that required fine-motor coordination. As a nurse, she suspected PD but did not accept the news until her condition had been officially diagnosed by her family doctor. Lucille feels that age and PD are equally to blame for her increasing fatigue and slowness. She leads an active life on their family farm, working in her garden, preparing full noon meals for the family, and helping her children with child care and light farmwork.

Marian is in her early sixties and caregiver to Stanley. She is a retired nurse, and she has been able to use her training to become a strong advocate for Stanley during doctors' visits and hospitalizations.

Martha is in her early sixties and is a full-time caregiver to her husband, Joe. Martha patiently cares for her ailing partner, lifting, bathing, dressing, and feeding him. She manages all their finances and housework and keeps track of his appointments and medications.

Mary is sixty and was diagnosed about ten years ago. Her PD is tremor dominant and she is prone to falling. Increasingly, her memory fails her and her voice is beginning to show signs of PD progression. Mary continues to work part-time, despite her impairments and fatigue, because of financial need. Her PD medications are a financial burden.

Mildred is a sixty-eight-year-old caregiver for her husband, Kenneth. She is an upbeat and energetic person who delights in gardening, housekeeping, and her family. She encourages Kenneth to stay active by dancing with him, reading him the paper, inviting the grandchildren over to visit, and taking daily walks on their land. Kenneth is slowly retreating inside himself as his communication problems grow more isolating, but Mildred persistently draws him out, giving him time to respond and asking him short directed questions. She recognizes that PD's progression is taking away her beloved partner and is doing her best to forestall the loss.

Oscar is seventy-two years old and has had PD for about six years. His first symptoms were cognitive, and it took quite a while for him to get a definitive diagnosis. He complains of "waviness" in the head and fatigue, and he cries easily. Oscar has an active calendar. Church, family, business, and volunteer activities keep him quite busy. The actions of other local support group members lead him to wonder if he should be taking a more aggressive stance toward his treatment. Oscar wonders if he should be seeking more specialized care and newer medications or remain with his current provider.

Peter was in his early eighties when we met and had had PD for more than five years. Peter's PD primarily affected his balance, coordination, and cognitive function. He had great difficulty putting words together into coherent phrases, and this communication issue dealt a sore blow to his self-confidence. Peter became increasingly reliant upon his wife, Laura, to speak for him and less inclined to participate in social activities. Less than a year after we met, Peter moved into a nursing home, where he passed away after an extended illness.

Ralph is eighty-one years old and has had PD for five years. His first and primary symptom was profound depression. Because of its severity and a family history of depression, Ralph sought treatment immediately. He was diagnosed with PD shortly thereafter. Ralph was retired when PD presented, and his symptoms do not interfere with his heavy volunteering schedule. He is an avid reader and author but has begun to refrain from attending social functions with his wife out of respect for her abilities. Ralph fears that he holds her back and sometimes prefers that she attend functions alone to better appreciate them.

Richard is seventy-seven years old and has had PD for ten years. He has a mild unilateral tremor and a slow, shuffling walk. He was forced to retire earlier than he had planned because he had difficulty remembering his trucking routes and customer information. Richard lives with his wife in their small country home and spends his days watching television and puttering in his shed. Richard has been plagued by hallucinations, and he and his wife have worked to find a reasonable balance between medicating enough so that he can function and using so much medication that he has disturbing visions. Richard's medication issues can be a source of sadness and frustration for his wife, who recently retired to care for him full-time.

Robert is seventy-four years old and lives with his wife, Sarah. He is semiretired from the clergy, an author, and volunteers in the community. He seems surprised that the PD has not had a greater effect on his life than it has, and confesses that he hadn't imagined that he could maintain an intimate relationship with his wife at his current age. Robert's faith and pragmatic nature mean that he approaches PD as something to be accepted and studied, but not as something that has to get in the way of your plans.

Rose is in her midseventies and widowed, and faces ongoing pressure from her family to leave her home and move into an assisted-living facility. She has a brother with PD and has herself lived with it for a decade. She is content in her little home and maintains an active social calendar. She has a winning and sharp sense of humor, which she often uses to deflect queries about her abilities.

Ruby is seventy-eight years old and has been living with PD for about ten years. She has moderate to severe tremor, postural instability, dyskinesia, and gait impairments. She and her husband remain snowbirds, traveling to Arizona for the long Iowa winters. There they have an active social life, surrounded by a community of similarly abled people. In Iowa, Ruby's life is a bit more constrained and she feels embarrassed by her shaking limbs.

Russell is seventy-nine years old and has had PD for seven years. His main symptoms are postural instability and hand tremor, but he has an emerging swallowing/speech problem and is diabetic. Russell has a full social calendar and continues to stay involved in his family business. He and his wife have been debating their snowbird behavior. Russell is adamant that they keep their property in the Southwest, but his wife is nervous about the long drive, the distance from familiar doctors, and the responsibility of selling it should one of them become seriously ill.

Sarah is a seventy-four-year-old caregiver to her husband, Robert. Sarah was the first person to recognize Robert's PD and asked him to see a doctor about his tremor and shuffling walk. Their Christian faith has helped them make sense of his PD and of her chronic illness. Sarah receives as much care as she gives, and together this couple manages to keep an immaculate house, participate in community organizations, and stay active members of their family.

Stanley is sixty-five years old and although he has only had PD for a few years, it has progressed quite rapidly. Stanley and his wife, Marian, have had to dramatically scale back their travel plans because of Stanley's disabilities. Once an avid runner and outdoor enthusiast, Stanley finds that his stamina and skills are sorely taxed by PD symptoms. He exercises daily to forestall further deterioration and maintains an optimistic outlook despite his surprise at the past few years' decline.

Thomas is in his midseventies and caregiver to Anna. Thomas is in good health and plans to care for Anna at home as long as possible. This role has meant that Thomas has had to give up recreational and social activities, and he is working hard to figure out how to manage the household and Anna's care at the same time. Adult day care has not been an acceptable option to Anna, and Thomas is exploring in-home respite services.

Vernon is in his mideighties and has had PD for less than a year. His moderate tremor is a source of great discomfort and embarrassment. Shaking hands are not consistent with his identity as a confident and capable businessman. Vernon strives to keep his PD under wraps and does not want to be pitied. However, he takes his situation seriously and changed physicians because he felt that his doctor did not give him the proper amount of attention.

Virginia is sixty-six years old and was fifty-nine when she was diagnosed with PD. Her first symptoms, slowness and an unsmiling expression, were noted by her family but didn't seem to Virginia to be anything of consequence. She finally decided that something was amiss when her once-beautiful penmanship began to deteriorate into the typical parkinsonian script—tiny block letters. Virginia and her husband recently decided to move from their two-story country farmhouse into a one-story ranch just outside town, in anticipation of her future limitations.

Wallace is in his early sixties and has severe PD. He has been unable to walk unassisted for several years and relies upon a motorized scooter for transportation. He recently had DBS surgery with little improvement and some worsening. His speech intelligibility increased but his motor function deteriorated further. Wallace had been working toward this surgery for several years and the lack of efficacy was a tremendous blow. He remains on high doses of PD medications to maintain his limited range of function.

APPENDIX B
SELECTED RESOURCES

U.S. Parkinson's Disease Advocacy Organizations

National Advocacy Organizations

American Parkinson's Disease Association
1250 Hylan Boulevard, Staten Island, NY 10305
Web Site: www.apdaparkinson.org

Bachmann-Strauss Dystonia and Parkinson Foundation, Inc.
One Gustave L. Levy Place, Box 1490, New York, NY 10029
Web Site: www.dystonia-parkinsons.org

Michael J. Fox Foundation for Parkinson's Research
20 Exchange Place, Suite 3200, New York, NY 10005
Web Site: www.michaeljfox.org

National Parkinson Foundation, Inc.
1501 N.W. Ninth Avenue, Miami, FL 33136
Web Site: www.parkinson.org

Parkinson Alliance
Post Office Box 308, Kingston, NJ 08528-0308
Web Site: www.parkinsonalliance.org

Parkinson's Action Network (PAN)
1025 Vermont Avenue NW, Suite 1120, Washington, DC 20005
Web Site: www.parkinsonsaction.org

Parkinson's Disease Foundation
1359 Broadway, Suite 1509, New York, NY 10018
Web Site: www.pdf.org

U.S. Regional Advocacy Organizations

Iowa Chapter of the American Parkinson's Disease Association
Web Site: www.apdaiowa.org/index.php

Northwest Parkinson's Foundation
P.O. Box 56, Mercer Island, WA 98040
Web Site: www.nwpf.org/

Parkinson Association of the Carolinas
601 E. Fifth Street, Suite 140, Charlotte, NC 28202 USA
Web Site: www.parkinsonassociation.org

Parkinson Foundation of the Heartland
7800 Foster, Overland Park, KS 66204-2955
Web Site: www.parkinsonheartland.org

Struther's Parkinson's Center
6701 Country Club Drive, Golden Valley, MN 55427
Web Site: www.parknicollet.com/Methodist/Parkinsons/

Wisconsin Parkinson's Association
945 N. Twelfth Street, Suite 4602, Milwaukee, WI 53233
Web Site: www.wiparkinson.org/

Young-Onset Organizations

Movers and Shakers Inc.
15275 Collier Boulevard, Suite 201, Box 151, Naples, FL 34119
Web Site: www.pdoutreach.org

Young Onset Parkinson's Association
111 Shawnee Loop N., Pataskala, OH 43062-8123
Web Site: www.yopa.org

Parkinson's Disease Narratives: Selected Bibliography

Aho, Kari. 2001. *Parkinson's Disease: My Constant Companion: A Neurologist's Experiences as a Patient.* Espoo, Finland: Anekdootti.

Anderson, Victor. 2006. *Carolyn's Journey: From Parkinson's Disease to a Nearly Normal Life after Deep Brain Stimulation.* Rogers, Minn.: DeForest Press.

Awalt, Jane Kriete. 2008. *The Stranger Comes at Sundown: Living and Dying with Parkinson's Disease.* Albuquerque: Rio Grande Books.

Dorros, Sidney. 1992. *Parkinson's: A Patient's View.* Santa Ana, Calif.: Seven Locks Press.

Fox, Michael J. 2002. *Lucky Man: A Memoir.* New York: Hyperion.

Gordon, Sandi. 1992. *Parkinson's: A Personal Story of Acceptance.* Boston: Branden.

Graboys, Thomas, and Peter Zheutlin. 2008. *Life in the Balance: A Physician's Memoir of Life, Love, and Loss with Parkinson's Disease and Dementia.* New York: Union Square Press.

Grady-Fitchett, Joan. 1998. *Flying Lessons: On the Wings of Parkinson's Disease.* New York: Forge.

Harshaw, William A. 2001. *My Second Life: Living with Parkinson's Disease.* Toronto: Tonawanda, N.Y.: Dundurn Press.

Havemann, Joel. 2002. *A Life Shaken: My Encounter with Parkinson's Disease*. Baltimore: Johns Hopkins University Press.

Jones, David. 2006. *Next to Me! Luck, Leadership, and Living with Parkinson's*. London: Nicholas Brealey.

Kondrake, Morton. 2001. *Saving Milly: Love, Politics, and Parkinson's Disease*. New York: PublicAffairs.

Layne, Bruce. 2003. *My Gift*. Las Vegas: Stephens Press.

Lightner, Patricia. 2003. *Parkinson's Disease and Me: Walking the Path*. N.p.: AuthorHouse.

Luscombe, Paul. 2006. *Pills, Bills, and Parkinson's Disease: Coping with the On and Off Syndrome*. Chatham, N.J.: PAL.

Morgan, Eric. 1997. *Defending against the Enemy: Coping with Parkinson's Disease*. Fort Bragg, Calif.: QED Press.

Newsom, Hal. 2002. *Hope: Four Keys to a Better Quality of Life for Parkinson's People*. Bellevue, Wash.: Northwest Parkinson's Foundation.

Popper, Eva B. 1988. *My Love, My Care, My Spouse: A Chronicle of Parkinson's Disease*. Beltsville, Md.: Parkinson Support Groups of America.

Todes, Cecil. 1990. *Shadow over My Brain: A Battle against Parkinson's Disease*. Moreton-in-Marsh, Gloucestershire: Windrush Press.

Vaughan, Ivan. 1987. *Ivan: Living with Parkinson's Disease*. New York: Farrar Straus and Giroux.

Webster, Kathleen. 2004. *Living with the Invisible Monster: A Young Onset Parkinson's Disease Patient's Perspective on Living a New Life*. N.p.: Authorhouse.

BIBLIOGRAPHY

Albert, Steven M. 2004. *Public Health and Aging: An Introduction to Maximizing Education and Well Being.* New York: Springer.

Albert, Steven M., and Maria Cattell. 1994. *Old Age in Global Perspective.* New York: Maxwell Macmillan International.

Alves, G., T. Wentzel-Larsen, D. Aarsland, and J. P. Larsen. 2005. Progression of motor impairment and disability in Parkinson disease: a population-based study. *Neurology* 65(9): 1436–1441.

Armstrong, M. J. 2005. Grandchildren's influences on grandparents: a resource for integration of older people in New Zealand's aging society. *Journal of Intergenerational Relationships: Programs, Policy, and Research* 3(2): 7–21.

Astin, John A., Kenneth R. Pelletier, Ariane Marie, and William L. Haskell. 2000. Complementary and alternative medicine use among elderly persons: a one-year analysis of a Blue Shield Medicare supplement. *Journals of Gerontology: Medical Sciences* 55A (I): M4–9.

Aujoulat, Isabelle, Olivier Luminet, and Alain Deccache. 2007. The perspective of patients on their experience of powerlessness. *Qualitative Health Research* 17(1): 772–785.

Baldi, I., P. Lebailly, B. Mohammed-Brahim, L. Letenneur, J.-F. Dartigues, and P. Brochard. 2003. Neurodegenerative diseases and exposure to pesticides in the elderly. *American Journal of Epidemiology* 157: 409–414.

Ball, M. M., M. M. Perkins, F. J. Whittington, C. Hollingsworth, S. V. King, and B. L. Combs. 2005. *Communities of Care: Assisted Living for African American Elders.* Baltimore: Johns Hopkins University Press.

Becker, Gay. 1997. *Disrupted Lives: How People Create Meaning in a Chaotic World.* Berkeley: University of California Press.

Behar, Ruth, and Deborah Gordon, eds. 1996. *Women Writing Culture.* Berkeley: University of California Press.

Berry, R. A., and J. F. Murphy. 1995. Well-being of caregivers of spouses with Parkinson's disease. *Clinical Nursing Research* 4(4): 373–386.

Birgersson, A. M., and A. K. Edberg. 2004. Being in the light or in the shade: persons with Parkinson's disease and their partners' experience of support. *International Journal of Nursing Studies* 41(6): 621–630.

Black, Helen K. 2006. *Soul Pain: The Meaning of Suffering in Later Life.* Society and Aging Series. Amityville, N.Y.: Baywood.

Black, Helen K., and Robert L. Rubinstein. 2000. *Old Souls: Aged Women, Poverty, and the Experience of God.* New York: A. de Gruyter.

———. 2004. Themes of suffering in later life. *Journals of Gerontology: Psychological Sciences and Social Sciences* 59(1): S17–S24.

Blumhagen, Dan W. 1981. On the nature of explanatory models. *Culture, Medicine, and Psychiatry* 5(4): 337–340.

Bond, Malcolm J., Michael S. Clark, and Suzanne Davies. 2003. The quality of life of spouse dementia caregivers: changes associated with yielding to formal care and widowhood. *Social Science and Medicine* 57: 2385–2395.

Bramley, N., and V. Eatough. 2005. The experience of living with Parkinson's disease: An interpretative phenomenological analysis case study. *Psychology and Health* 20(2): 223–235.

Brod, M., G. A. Mendelsohn, and B. Roberts. 1998. Patients' experience of Parkinson's disease. *Journals of Gerontology: Psychological Sciences and Social Sciences* 53B (4): 213–222.

Brown, T. P., P. C. Rumsby, A. C. Capleton, L. Rushton, and L. S. Levy. 2006. Pesticides and Parkinson's disease—is there a link? *Environmental Health Perspectives* 114: 156–164.

Bury, Michael. 1982. Chronic illness as biographical disruption. *Sociology of Health and Illness* 4: 165–182.

Caap-Ahlgren, M., L. Lannerheim, and O. Dehlin. 2002. Older Swedish women's experiences of living with symptoms related to Parkinson's disease. *Journal of Advanced Nursing* 39(1): 87–95.

Charlton, G. S., and C. J. Barrow. 2002. Coping and self-help group membership in Parkinson's disease: an exploratory qualitative study. *Health and Social Care in the Community* 10(6): 472–478.

Charmaz, Kathy. 1983. Loss of self: a fundamental form of suffering in the chronically ill. *Sociology of Health and Illness* 5(2): 168–195.

———. 1991. *Good Days, Bad Days: Illness and Time.* New Brunswick, N.J.: Rutgers University Press.

Chibnik, Michael. 1985. The use of statistics in sociocultural anthropology. *Annual Review of Anthropology* 14: 135–157.

Chrischilles, Elizabeth A., Linda M. Rubenstein, Margaret D. Voelker, Robert B. Wallace, and Robert L. Rodnitzsky. 1998. The health burdens of Parkinson's disease. *Movement Disorders* 13(3): 406–413.

Chung, Joseph S., Allan D. Wu, and Mark F. Lew. 2003. Amantadine and anticholinergics. In *Handbook of Parkinson's Disease*, ed. R. Pahwa, K. E. Lyons, and W. C. Koller. New York: Marcel Dekker.

Cliggett, Lisa. 2005. *Grains from Grass: Aging, Gender, and Famine in Rural Africa.* Ithaca, N.Y.: Cornell University Press.

Cohen, Lawrence. 1994. Old age: cultural and critical perspectives. *Annual Reviews in Anthropology* 23(1): 137–158.

Conley, Scott C., and Jeffrey T. Kirchner. 1999. Medical and surgical treatment of Parkinson's disease. *Postgraduate Medicine* 106(2): 41–52.

Conrad, Peter. 1990. Qualitative research on chronic illness: A commentary on method and conceptual development. *Social Science and Medicine* 30(11): 1257–1263.

Corbin, Juliet M. 2003. The body in health and illness. *Qualitative Health Research* 13(2): 256–267.

Corbin, Juliet M., and Anselm Strauss. 1988. *Unending Work and Care: Managing Chronic Illness at Home.* San Francisco: Jossey-Bass.

Crawford, Robert. 1984. A cultural account of "health": control, release, and the social body. In *Issues in the Political Economy of Health Care*, ed. J. B. McKinlay. New York: Tavistock.

Crews, Douglas E. 2003. *Human Senescence: Evolutionary and Biocultural Perspectives.* Cambridge Studies in Biological and Evolutionary Anthropology. Cambridge: Cambridge University Press.

Csordas, Thomas J. 1990. Embodiment as a paradigm for anthropology. *Ethos* 18(1): 5–47.

———. 1993a. Introduction: The body as representation and being-in-the-world. In *Embodiment and Experience: The Existential Ground of Culture and Self*, ed. T. J. Csordas. New York: Cambridge University Press.

———. 1993b. Somatic modes of attention. *Cultural Anthropology* 8(2): 135–156.

———. 2002. *Body/Meaning/Healing*. 1st ed. Contemporary Anthropology of Religion. New York: Palgrave Macmillan.

Curtis, Robin, and Sylvia McDonald. 1998. Alterations in motor function. In *Pathophysiology: Concepts of Altered Health States*, ed. C. M. Porth. 5th ed. Philadelphia: Lippincott.

Davis-Floyd, Robbie. 2003. *Birth As an American Rite of Passage*. 2nd ed. Berkeley: University of California Press.

Dewey, Richard B. 2003. Nonmotor symptoms of Parkinson's disease. In *Handbook of Parkinson's Disease*, ed. R. Pahwa, K. E. Lyons, and W. C. Koller. New York: Marcel Dekker.

Douglas, Mary. 1966. *Purity and Danger: An Analysis of Concepts of Pollution and Taboo*. New York: Praeger.

Duvoisin, Roger C., and Jacob Sage. 1996. *Parkinson's Disease: A Guide for Patient and Family*. 4th ed. Philadelphia: Lippincott-Raven.

Edwards, Nancy E. 2002. The influence of caregiver burden on patients' management of Parkinson's disease: implications for rehabilitation nursing. *Rehabilitation Nursing* 27(5): 182–186.

Eisenberg, Leon. 1977. Diseases and illness: distinctions between professional and popular ideas of sickness. *Culture, Medicine, and Psychiatry* 1(1): 9–23.

Epstein, Steven. 1999. The construction of lay expertise: AIDS activism and the forging of credibility in the reform of clinical trials. *Science, Technology, and Human Values* 20(4): 408–437.

Faircloth, Christopher A., ed. 2003a. *Aging Bodies: Images and Everyday Experience*. Walnut Creek, Calif.: Altamira Press.

———. 2003b. Different bodies and the paradox of aging: locating bodies in images and everyday experience. In *Aging Bodies: Images and Everyday Experience*, ed. C. A. Faircloth. Walnut Creek, Calif.: Altamira Press.

Faircloth, Christopher A., Craig Boylstein, Maude Rittman, and Mary Ellen Young. 2004. Disrupted bodies: experiencing the newly limited body in stroke. *Symbolic Interaction* 27(1) : 71–87.

Farmer, Paul, and Byron J. Good. 1991. Illness representations in medical anthropology: a critical review and a case study of the representation of AIDS in Haiti. In *Mental Representation in Health and Illness*, ed. J. A. Skelton and R. T. Croyle. New York: Springer-Verlag.

Farrer, M. J. 2006. Genetics of Parkinson disease: paradigm shifts and future prospects. *Nature* 7: 306–318.

FEDSTATS 2008. Source: Bureau of Economic Analysis, Bureau of Labor Statistics, National Agricultural Statistics Service, National Center for Health Statistics, U.S. Census Bureau. Last revised: 14 April 2008. www.fedstats.gov/qf/states/19000.html.

Fernandez, Hubert H., Rowena E. J. Tabamo, Raymund R. David, and Joseph H. Friedman. 2001. Predictors of depressive symptoms among spouse caregivers in Parkinson's disease. *Movement Disorders* 16(6): 1123–1125.

Fink, H. A., M. A. Kuskowski, E. S. Orwoll, J. A. Cauley, and K. E. Ensrud. 2005. Association between Parkinson's disease and low bone density and falls in older men: The Osteoporotic Fractures in Men study. *Journal of the American Geriatrics Society* 53(9): 1559–1564.

Finkler, Kaja. 1994. *Women in Pain: Gender and Morbidity in Mexico*. Philadelphia: University of Pennsylvania Press.

Fischer, P. 1999. Parkinson's disease and the U.S. health care system. *Journal of Community Health Nursing* 16(3): 191–204.

Fitzsimmons, B., and L. K. Bunting. 1993. Parkinson's disease: quality of life issues. *Nursing Clinics of North America* 28(4): 807–818.

Fleming, V., D. Tolson, and E. Schartau. 2004. Changing perceptions of womanhood: living with Parkinson's disease. *International Journal of Nursing Studies* 41(5): 515–524.

Foltynie, Thomas, Carol Brayne, and Roger A. Barker. 2002. The heterogeneity of idiopathic Parkinson's disease. *Journal of Neurology* 249: 138–145.

Foster, George M., and Barbara Gallatin Anderson. 1978. *Medical Anthropology*. New York: John Wiley and Sons.

Francis, Doris, Leonie A. Kellaher, and Georgina Neophytou. 2005. *The Secret Cemetery*. New York: Berg.

Frank, Arthur W. 2001. Can we research suffering? *Qualitative Health Research* 11(3): 353–362.

Friesen, Ingrid, and Catherine A. Mateer. 2001. Memory and executive dysfunction in elderly people: the role of the frontal lobes. In *Behavioral Neurology in the Elderly*, ed. J. Leon-Carrion, and Margaret J. Giannini. New York: CRC Press.

Fry, Christine L. 1980. Toward an anthropology of aging. In *Aging in Culture and Society: Comparative Viewpoints and Strategies*, ed. C. L. Fry. New York: J. F. Bergin.

———. 2006. When age becomes irrelevant: The mystery of cross-age relationships. *Anthropology and Aging Quarterly* 27(2): 8–11, 35.

Fuller, George F. 1997. Falls in the elderly. *American Family Physician* 58: 1815–1823.

Gerhardt, Uta. 1990. Qualitative research in chronic illness: the issue and the story. *Social Science and Medicine* 30(11): 1149–1159.

Golbe, L. I., G. Di Iorio, A. Lazzarini, P. Vieregge, O. S. Gershanik, V. Bonavita,, and C. R. Duvoisin.1999. The Contursi kindred, a large family with autosomal dominant Parkinson's disease: implications of clinical and molecular studies. In *Advances in Neurology*, vol. 80, *Parkinson's Disease*, ed. G Stern, 165–170. New York: Lippincott Williams and Wilkins.

Good, Byron J. 1994. *Medicine, Rationality, and Experience: An Anthropological Perspective*. New York: Cambridge University Press.

Gubrium, Jaber F., and James A. Holstein. 1999. Constructionist perspectives on aging. In *Handbook of Theories of Aging*, ed. V. L. Bengston and K. W. Schaie. New York: Springer.

———. 2003. The everyday visibility of the aging body. In *Aging Bodies: Images and Everyday Experience*, ed. C. A. Faircloth. Walnut Creek, Calif.: Altamira Press.

Gullette, Margaret Morganroth. 2004. *Aged by Culture*. Chicago: University of Chicago Press.

Herskovits, Elizabeth. 1995. Struggling over subjectivity: debates about the "self" and Alzheimer's disease. *Medical Anthropology Quarterly* 9(2): 146–164.

Hockey, Jenny, and Allison James. 2003. *Social Identities across the Life Course*. New York: Palgrave Macmillan.

Hoehn, M. M., and M. D. Yahr. 1967. Parkinsonism: onset, progression, and mortality. *Neurology* 17(5): 427–442.

Hopfensburger, K., and W. C. Keller. 1991. Recognizing early Parkinson's disease. *Postgraduate Medicine* 90: 49–50, 5–6, 9.

Iansek, Robert. 1999. Interdisciplinary rehabilitation in Parkinson's disease. In *Advances in Neurology*, vol. 80, *Parkinson's Disease*, ed. G. Stern. New York: Lippincott Williams and Wilkins.

Ice, Gillian. 2005. Biological anthropology and aging. *Journal of Crosscultural Gerontology* 20(2): 87–90.

IDALS 2006. Facts about Iowa Agriculture. Des Moines, Iowa: Iowa Department of Agriculture and Land Stewardship. www.agriculture.state.ia.us/agfacts.htm.

IDEA 2006. *Older Iowans* 2006. Des Moines, Iowa: Iowa Department of Elder Affairs. www.iowadatacenter.org/Publications/OlderIowans/.

Iezzoni, Lisa I. 2003. *When Walking Fails: Mobility Problems of Adults with Chronic Conditions.* Berkeley: University of California Press.

Ingadottir, Brynja, and Sigridur Halldorsdottir. 2008. To discipline a "dog": the essential structure of mastering diabetes. *Qualitative Health Research* 18(5): 606–619.

Ironside, P. M., M. Scheckel, C. Wessels, M. E. Bailey, S. Powers, and D. K. Seeley. 2003. Experiencing chronic illness: cocreating new understandings. *Qualitative Health Research* 13(2): 171–183.

Jankovic, Joseph. 2003. Pathophysiology and clinical assessment of parkinsonism symptoms and signs. In *Handbook of Parkinson's Disease*, ed. R. Pahwa, K. E. Lyons, and W. C. Koller. New York: Marcel Dekker.

Jenkinson, C., R. Fitzpatrick, and V. Peto. 1999. Health-related quality-of-life measurement in patients with Parkinson's disease. *Pharmacoeconomics* 15: 157–165.

Jervis, Lori L. 2001. The pollution of incontinence and the dirty work of caregiving in a U.S. nursing home. *Medical Anthropology Quarterly* 15(1): 84–99.

Kaufman, Sharon. 1988. Toward a phenomenology of boundaries in medicine: chronic illness experience in the case of stroke. *Medical Anthropology Quarterly* 2(4): 338.

Keith, Jennie. 1980. "The best is yet to be": toward an anthropology of age. *Annual Reviews in Anthropology* 9: 339–364.

Keith, Jennie, and David I. Kertzer. 1984. Introduction to *Age and Anthropological Theory*, ed. D. I. Kertzer and J. Keith. Ithaca, N.Y.: Cornell University Press.

Kelley, Mary Lou, and Michael J. MacLean. 1997. I want to live here for the rest of my life: the challenge of case management for rural seniors. *Journal of Case Management* 6(4): 174–182.

Kirschstein, Ruth L. 2000. *Parkinson's Disease Research Agenda.* Washington D.C.: National Institute of Neurological Disorders and Stroke.

Kleinman, Arthur. 1977. Rethinking the social and cultural context of psychopathology and psychiatric care. In *Renewal Psychiatry: A Critical Rational Perspective*, ed. T. C. Manschreck and A. Kleinman. New York: John Wiley and Sons.

——. 1978. Concepts and a model for the comparison of medical systems as cultural systems. *Social Science and Medicine* 12: 85–93.

——. 1981. On illness meanings and cultural interpretation: not "rational man," but a rational approach to man the sufferer/man the healer. *Culture, Medicine, and Psychiatry* 5(4): 373–377.

——. 1988a. *The Illness Narratives.* New York: Basic Books.

——. 1988b. *Rethinking Psychiatry: From Cultural Category to Personal Experience.* New York: The Free Press.

Kleinman, Arthur, Veena Das, and Margaret Lock. 1996. Social suffering—introduction. *Daedalus* 125(1): R11–R20.

——. 1997. *Social suffering.* Berkeley: University of California Press.

Koenig, Barbara A., and Patricia Marshall. 2004. Anthropology and bioethics. In *Encyclopedia of Bioethics*, ed. S. Post. 3rd ed. New York: Macmillan.

Koller, W., B. Vetere-Overfield, C. Gray, S. Alexander, T. Chin, and J. Dolezal. 1990. Environmental risk factors in Parkinson's disease. *Neurology* 40: 1218–1221.

Koplas, P.A., H. P. Gans, M. P. Wisely, M. Kuchibhatla, T. M. Cutson, D. T. Gold, C. T. Taylor, and M. Schenkman. 1999. Quality of life and Parkinson's disease. *Journals of Gerontology: Biological Sciences and Medical Sciences* 54A(4): M 197–202.

Kramer, Betty J. 1997. Gain in the caregiving experience: Where are we? What next? *The Gerontologist* 31(2): 218–232.

Krout, J. A. 1994. An overview of older rural populations and community-based services. In *Providing Community-Based Services to the Rural Elderly*, ed. J. A. Krout, 3–18. Thousand Oaks, Calif.: Sage Publications.

———. 1997. Barriers to providing case management to older rural persons. *Journal of Case Management* 6(4): 142–150.

Krout, J. A., and R. T. Coward, eds. 1998. *Aging in Rural Settings: Life Circumstances and Distinctive Features.* New York: Springer.

Kunstadter, Peter. 1974. The comparative anthropological study of medical systems in society. In *Medicine in Chinese Cultures: Comparative Studies of Health Care in Chinese and Other Societies*, ed. A. Kleinman, P. Kunstadter, A. E. Russell, and J. E. Gale. Washington, D.C.: National Institutes of Health, U.S. Government Printing Office.

Kuopio, A. M., R. J. Marttila, H. Helenius, and U. K. Rinne. 1999. Environmental risk factors in Parkinson's disease. *Movement Disorders* 14(6): 928–939.

Lang, A.E., and A. M. Lozano. 1998a. Parkinson's disease: first of two parts. *New England Journal of Medicine* 339(15): 1044–1053.

———. 1998b. Parkinson's disease: second of two parts. *New England Journal of Medicine* 339(16): 1130–1143.

Latour, Bruno. 2000. When things strike back: a possible contribution of "science studies" to the social sciences. *British Journal of Sociology* 51(1): 107–123.

Laz, Cheryl. 2003. Age embodied. *Journal of Aging Studies* 17: 503–519.

Le Couteur, D. G., A. J. McLean, M. C. Taylor, B. L. Woodham, and P. G. Board. 1999. Pesticides and Parkinson's disease. *Biomedicine and Pharmacotherapy* 53: 122–130.

LeDuff, Charlie. 2003. Eight die after driver plows through outdoor California market. *New York Times*, July 17.

Leibing, Annette, and Lawrence Cohen. 2006. *Thinking about Dementia: Culture, Loss, and the Anthropology of Senility, Studies in Medical Anthropology.* New Brunswick, N.J.: Rutgers University Press.

Leibing, Annette, and Athena McLean. 2007. "Learn to value your shadow!" an introduction to the margins of fieldwork. In *The Shadow Side of Fieldwork: Exploring the Blurred Borders between Ethnography and Life*, ed. Ethan McLean and Annette Leibing. Malden, Mass.: Blackwell.

Le Navenec, Carole-Lynne, and Laurel Bridges. 2005. *Creating Connections between Nursing Care and the Creative Arts Therapies: Expanding the Concept of Holistic Care.* Springfield, Ill.: Charles C. Thomas.

Lewis, S.J.G., T. Foltynie, A. D. Blackwell, T. W. Robbins, A. M. Owen, and R. A. Barker. 2005. Heterogeneity of Parkinson's disease in the early clinical stages using a data driven approach. *Journal of Neurology, Neurosurgery, and Psychiatry* 76(3): 343–348.

Lieberman, Abraham. 2002. *Shaking Up Parkinson's Disease: Fighting Like a Tiger, Thinking Like a Fox.* Sudbury, Mass.: Jones and Bartlett.

Lilley, J. M., T. Arie, and C.E.D. Chilvers. 1995. Special review: accidents involving older people: a review of the literature. *Age and Ageing* 24: 346–365.

Lindgren, Carolyn L. 1996. Chronic sorrow in persons with Parkinson's and their spouses. *Scholarly Inquiry for Nursing Practice: An International Journal* 10(4): 351–370.

Liou, H. H., M. C. Tsia, C. J. Chen, J. S. Jeng, Y. C. Chang, S. Y. Chen, and R. C. Chen. 1997. Environmental risk factors and Parkinson's disease: a case-control study in Taiwan. *Neurology* 48: 1583–1588.

Lock, Margaret. 1993. Cultivating the body: anthropology and epistemologies of bodily practice and knowledge. *Annual Review of Anthropology* 22: 133–155.

Lupton, Deborah. 1994. *Medicine as Culture: Illness, Disease, and the Body in Western Societies.* Thousand Oaks, Calif.: Sage Publications.

Lyons, K. S., B. J. Stewart, P. G. Archbold, J. H. Carter, and N. A. Perrin. 2004. Pessimism and optimism as early warning signs for compromised health for caregivers of patients with Parkinson's disease. *Nursing Research* 53(6): 354–362.

Manyam, Bala V., and Juan R. Sanchez-Ramos. 1999. Traditional and complementary therapies in Parkinson's disease. In *Advances in Neurology*, vol. 80, *Parkinson's Disease*, ed. G. Stern. New York: Lippincott Williams and Wilkins.

Marcus, George E. 1998. Ethnography in/of the world system: the emergence of multi-sited ethnography. In *Ethnography through Thick and Thin*, ed. G. E. Marcus. Princeton, N.J.: Princeton University Press.

Marder, K., G. Logroscino, B. Alfaro, H. Mejia, A. Halim, E. Louis, L. Cote, and R. Mayeux. 1998. Environmental risk factors for Parkinson's disease in an urban multiethnic community. *Neurology* 50: 279–281.

Martin, Emily. 1987. *The Woman in the Body: A Cultural Analysis of Reproduction.* Boston: Beacon Press.

———. 1997. Anthropology and the cultural study of science: from citadels to string figures. In *Anthropological Locations: Boundaries and Grounds of Field Science*, ed. A. Gupta and J. Ferguson. Berkeley: University of California Press.

Mattingly, Cheryl. 1998. *Healing Dramas and Clinical Plots.* New York: Cambridge University Press.

McLaughlin, Diane K., and Leif Jensen. 1998. The rural elderly: a demographic portrait. In *Aging in Rural Settings: Life Circumstances and Distinctive Features*, ed. R. T. Coward and J. A. Krout. New York: Springer.

McLean, Athena. 2006. *The Person in Dementia.* Orchard Park, N.Y.: Broadview Press.

McRae, C., P. Sherry, and K. Roper. 1999. Stress and family functioning among caregivers of persons with Parkinson's disease. *Parkinsonism and Related Disorders* 5(1–2): 69–75.

Meara, Jolyon. 2000. A glossary of terms. In *Parkinson's Disease and Parkinsonism in the Elderly*, ed. J. Meara and W. C. Koller. New York: Cambridge University Press.

Meara, Jolyon, and Bimal K. Bhowmick. 2000. Parkinson's disease and parkinsonism in the elderly. In *Parkinson's Disease and Parkinsonism in the Elderly*, ed. J. Meara and W. C. Koller. New York: Cambridge University Press.

Meara, Jolyon, and Peter Hobson 2000. The epidemiology of Parkinson's disease and parkinsonism in elderly subjects. In *Parkinson's Disease and Parkinsonism in the Elderly*, ed. Meara and W. C. Koller New York: Cambridge University Press.

Mendehlson, Everett. 1974. Comparative studies in science and medicine: problems and perspectives. In *Medicine in Chinese Cultures: Comparative Studies of Health Care in Chinese and Other Societies*, ed. A. Kleinman, P. Kunstadter, E. R. Alexander, and J. E. Gale. Washington, D.C.: National Institutes of Health, U.S. Government Printing Office.

Mizuno, Y., S. Shimoda-Matsubayashi, H. Matsumine, N. Morikawa, N. Hattori, and T. Kondo. 1999. Genetic and environmental factors in the pathogenesis of Parkinson's disease. In *Advances in Neurology*, vol. 80, *Parkinson's Disease*, ed. G Stern, 171–180. New York: Lippincott Williams and Wilkins.

Mockenhaupt, Robin E., and Jennifer A. Muchow. 1994. Disease and disability prevention and health promotion for rural elders. In *Providing Community-Based Services to the Rural Elderly*, ed. J. A. Krout. Thousand Oaks, Calif.: Sage Publications.

Moerman, Daniel E. 2002. *Meaning, Medicine, and the "Placebo Effect."* Cambridge Studies in Medical Anthropology. Cambridge; New York: Cambridge University Press.

Monguio, Ines. 2001. Emotional disorders in the neurologically deteriorating older adult. In *Behavioral Neurology in the Elderly*, ed. J. Leon-Carrion and M. J. Giannini. New York: CRC Press.

Monks, Judith, and Ronald Frankenberg. 1995. Being ill and being me: Self, body, and time in multiple sclerosis narratives. In *Disability and Culture*, ed. B. Ingstad and Susan Reynolds-Whyte. Berkeley: University of California Press.

Murray, C. D., and B. Harrison. 2004. The meaning and experience of being a stroke survivor: an interpretative phenomenological analysis. *Disability and Rehabilitation* 26(13): 808–816.

Myerhoff, Barbara G. 1978. Aging and the aged in other cultures: an anthropological perspective. In *Anthropology of Health*, ed. E. E. Bauwens. St. Louis: C. V. Mosby.

Myerhoff, Barbara G., and Andrei Simic, eds. 1978. *Life's Career—Aging: Cultural Variations on Growing Old*. Beverly Hills, Calif.: Sage Publications.

Nader, Laura 1972. Up the anthropologist: perspectives gained from studying up. In *Reinventing Anthropology*, ed. Dell H. Hymes. New York: Pantheon Books.

Narayan, Kirin. 1993. How native is a "native" anthropologist? *American Anthropologist* 95(3): 671–686.

National Center for Injury Prevention and Control. 2001. Injury Fact Book 2001–2002. Atlanta, GA: Centers for Disease Control and Prevention.

Nijhof, Gerhard. 1995. Parkinson's disease as a problem of shame in public appearance. *Sociology of Health and Illness* 17(2): 193–205.

National Institute of Neurological Disorders and Stroke. 2000. *Parkinson's Disease Backgrounder*. Washington, D.C.: National Institutes of Health, U.S. Government Printing Office.

Noonan, Anne E., and Sharon L. Tennstedt. 1997. Meaning in caregiving and its contribution to caregiver well-being. *The Gerontologist* 37(6): 785–794.

Ohman M, S. Soderberg, and B. Lundman. 2003. Hovering between suffering and enduring: the meaning of living with serious chronic illness. *Qualitative Health Research* 13(4): 528–542.

Ono, Sarah. 2001. Peeling back tinsel: An anthropologist in Hollywood. Master's thesis, Department of Anthropology, University of Iowa.

O'Reilly, Fiona, F. Finnan, S. Allwright, G. D. Smith, and Yoav Ben-Shlomo. 1996. The effects of caring for a spouse with Parkinson's disease on social, psychological, and physical well-being. *British Journal of General Practice* 46: 507–512.

Pahwa, Rajesh, and Kelly E. Lyons. 2003. Deep brain stimulation in Parkinson's disease. In *Handbook of Parkinson's Disease*, ed. R. Pahwa, K. E. Lyons, and W. C. Koller. New York: Marcel Dekker.

Parker, M., J. Quinn, M. Viehl, A. H. McKinley, C. L. Polich, S. Hartwell, R. Van Hook, and D. F. Detzner. 1992. Issues in rural case management. *Family and Community Health* 14(4): 40–60.

Parsons, Talcott. 1979. Definitions of health and illness in the light of American values and social structure. In *Patients, Physicians, and Illness*, ed. E. G. Jaco. New York: Free Press.

Pfeiffer, Ronald F. 2003. Catechol-o-methyltransferase in Parkinson's disease. In *Handbook of Parkinson's Disease*, ed. R. Pahwa, K. E. Lyons, and W. C. Koller. New York: Marcel Dekker.

Pierret, Janine. 2003. The illness experience: state of knowledge and perspectives for research. *Sociology of Health and Illness* 25(3): 4–22.

Pinder, Ruth. 1990. *The Management of Chronic Illness: Patient and Doctor Perspectives on Parkinson's Disease.* Hong Kong: Macmillan.

———. 1992. Coherence and incoherence: doctors' and patients' perspectives on the diagnosis of Parkinson's disease. *Sociology of Health and Illness* 14(1): 1–22.

Priyadarshi, A., S. A. Khuder, E. A. Schaub, and S. Shrivastava. 2000. A meta-analysis of Parkinson's disease and exposure to pesticides. *Neurotoxicology* 21: 435–440.

Rajendran, P. R., R. E. Thompson, and S. G. Reich. 2001. The use of alternative therapies by patients with Parkinson's disease. *Neurology* 57(5): 790–794.

Rajput, Ali H., Alex Rajput, and Michele Rajput. 2003. Epidemiology of parkinsonism. In *Handbook of Parkinson's Disease*, ed. R. Pahwa, K. E. Lyons, and W. C. Koller. New York: Marcel Dekker.

RAND Corporation. 2006. *MOS* 36-Item Short Form Survey Instrument (SF-36). Retrieved April 2007 at www.rand.org/health/surveys_tools/mos/mos_core_36item.html.

Redford, Linda J., and Nancy L. Severns. 1994. Home health services in rural America. In *Providing Community-Based Services to the Rural Elderly*, ed. J. A. Krout. Thousand Oaks, Calif.: Sage Publications.

Reynolds, Frances, and Sarah Prior. 2003. "Sticking jewels in your life": exploring women's strategies for negotiating an acceptable quality of life with multiple sclerosis. *Qualitative Health Research* 13(9): 1225–1251.

Richards, L. 1999. Computer monitor: data alive! the thinking behind NVivo. *Qualitative Health Research* 9(3): 412–428.

Riessman, Catherine Kohler. 1993. *Narrative Analysis.* Qualitative Research Methods Series 30. Newbury Park, Calif.: Sage Publications.

———. 2001. Performing identities in illness narrative: masculinity and multiple sclerosis. Paper read at British Medical Association Conference, "Narrative-Based Medicine," Homerton College, Cambridge, U.K.

Rodnitzsky, Robert L. 2000. Diagnosis of parkinsonism in the elderly. In *Parkinson's Disease and Parkinsonism in the Elderly*, ed. J. Meara and W. C. Koller. New York: Cambridge University Press.

Romanucci-Ross, Lola, Danielle E. Moerman, and Laurence R. Tancredi. 1991. "Medical anthropology": convergence of mind and experience in the anthropological imagination. In *The Anthropology of Medicine: From Culture to Method*, ed. L. Romanucci-Ross, J. Monks, and L. R. Tancredi. New York: Bergin and Garvey.

Rowe, John W., and Robert L. Kahn 1998. *Successful Aging* New York: Pantheon Books.

Rubenstein, Linda M., Elizabeth A. Chrischilles, and Margaret D. Voelker. 1997. The impact of Parkinson's disease on health status, health expenditures, and productivity. *Pharmacoeconomics* 12: 486–498.

Rubenstein, Linda M., Andrea DeLeo, and Elizabeth A. Chrischilles. 2001. Economic and health-related quality of life: considerations of new therapies in Parkinson's disease. *Pharmacoeconomics* 19: 729–752.

Samuel, Michael, and Anthony E. Lang. 2003. Lesion surgeries. In *Handbook of Parkinson's disease*, ed. R. Pahwa, K. E. Lyons, and W. C. Koller. New York: Marcel Dekker.

Sato, Y., M. Kaji, T. Tsuru, and K. Oizumi. 2001. Risk factors for hip fracture among elderly patients with Parkinson's disease. *Journal of the Neurological Sciences* 182(2): 89–93.

Sato, Y., M. Kikuyama, and K. Oizumi. 1997. High prevalence of vitamin D deficiency and reduced bone mass in Parkinson's disease. *Neurology* 49(5): 1273–1278.

Savishinsky, Joel S. 2000. *Breaking the Watch: The Meanings of Retirement in America.* Ithaca, N.Y.: Cornell University Press.

Scheper-Hughes, Nancy, and Margaret M. Lock. 1987. The mindful body: A prolegomenon to future work in medical anthropology. *Medical Anthropology Quarterly* 1(1): 6–41.

Schoenfelder, D. P., and K. V. Why. 1997. A fall prevention educational program for community-dwelling seniors. *Public Health Nursing* 14: 383–390.

Schrag, Anette. 2004. Psychiatric aspects of Parkinson's disease: an update. *Journal of Neurology* 251: 795–804.

Schreurs, K.M.G., D.T.D. De Ridder, and J. M. Bensing. 2000. A one-year study of coping, social support, and quality of life in Parkinson's disease. *Psychology and Health* 15(1): 109–121.

Sethi, Kapil D. 2003. Differential diagnosis of parkinsonism. In *Handbook of Parkinson's Disease*, ed. R. Pahwa, K. E. Lyons, and W. C. Koller. New York: Marcel Dekker.

Settersten, Richard A., Jr. 2003. *Invitation to the Life Course: Toward New Understandings of Later Life*. Amityville, N.Y.: Baywood.

Shenk, Dena. 1998. Subjective realities of older women's lives: a case study. In *Old, Female, and Rural*, ed. B. J. McCulloch, 7–24. New York: Haworth Press.

Shortell, Stephen M., Robin R. Gillies, David A. Anderson, Karen Morgan Erickson, and John B. Mitchell. 2000. *Remaking Health Care in America: The Evolution of Organized Delivery Systems*. San Francisco: Jossey-Bass.

Simmons, Leo W. 1945. *The Role of the Aged in Primitive Society*. New Haven; London: Yale University Press; H. Milford, Oxford University Press.

Singh, Asha, Geetha Kandimala, Richard B. Dewey Jr., and Padraig O'Suilleanhain. 2007. Risk factors for pathologic gambling and other compulsions among Parkinson's disease patients taking dopamine agonists. *Journal of Clinical Neuroscience* 14(12): 1178–1181.

Solimeo, Samantha. 2008. Sex and gender in older adults' experience of Parkinson's disease. *Journals of Gerontology, Series B, Social Sciences* 63: S42–S48

Stacy, Mark A. 2003. Dopamine agonists. In *Handbook of Parkinson's Disease*, ed. R. Pahwa, K. E. Lyons, and W. C. Koller. New York: Marcel Dekker.

Stafford, Philip B. 2003. *Gray Areas: Ethnographic Encounters with Nursing Home Culture*. 1st ed. School of American Research Advanced Seminar Series. Santa Fe; Oxford: School of American Research Press; James Currey.

Staiano, Kathryn Vance. 1986. *Interpreting Signs of Illness: A Case Study in Medical Semiotics*. New York: Mouton de Gruyter.

Stamm, Tanja, Linda Lovelock, Graham Stew, Valeria Nell, Josef Smolen, Hans Jonsson, Gaynor Sadlo, and Klaus Maschold. 2008. I have mastered the challenge of living with a chronic disease: life stories of people with rheumatoid arthritis. *Qualitative Health Research* 18(5): 659–669.

Starkstein, Sergio E., and Marcelo Merello. 2002. *Psychiatric and Cognitive Disorders in Parkinson's Disease*. New York: Cambridge University Press.

Stein, Howard F. 1990. *American Medicine as Culture*. Boulder, Colo.: Westview Press.

Strathern, Marilyn. 2004. The whole person and its artifacts. *Annual Review of Anthropology* 33: 1–19.

Strauss, Anselm L., and Juliet Corbin. 1984. *Chronic Illness and the Quality of Life*. St. Louis: C. V. Mosby.

Svenaeus, F. 2000. The body uncanny—further steps towards a phenomenology of illness. *Medicine, Health Care, and Philosophy* 3(2): 125–137.

Tanner, Caroline M., and Yoav Ben-Shlomo. 1999. Epidemiology of Parkinson's disease. In *Advances in Neurology*, vol. 80, *Parkinson's Disease*, ed. G. Stern. New York: Lippincott Williams and Wilkins.

Taussig, Michael T. 1980. Reification and the consciousness of the patient. *Social Science and Medicine* 14B (2): 3–13.

Tedlock, Barbara. 1991. From participant observation to the observation of participation: the emergence of narrative ethnography. *Journal of Anthropological Research* 47(1): 69–94.

Thomas, S., and A. Dick. 1998. Parkinson's disease: overview of the disease and its treatment. *Elderly Care* 10(6): 39–40, 42.

Tickle-Degnen, Linda, and Kathleen Doyle Lyons. 2004. Practitioners' impressions of patients with Parkinson's disease: the social ecology of the expressive mask. *Social Science and Medicine* 58: 603–614.

Tinetti, M. 1994. Prevention of falls and fall injuries in elderly persons: a research agenda. *Preventive Medicine* 23: 756–762.

Tuchsen, F., and A. A. Jensen. 2000. Agricultural work and the risk of Parkinson's disease in Denmark, 1981–1993. *Scandinavian Journal of Work, Environment, and Health* 26: 359–362.

Turner, Terrence. 1993. Bodies and anti-bodies: flesh and fetish in contemporary social theory. In *Embodiment and Experience: The Existential Ground of Culture and Self*, ed. T. J. Csordas. New York: Cambridge University Press.

U.S. Census Bureau. 2000a. DP-1. Profile of General Demographic Characteristics: 2000. Geographic Area: Iowa. Vol. 2003. Washington, D.C.: U.S. Census Bureau.

———. 2000b. DP-2. Profile of Selected Social Characteristics: 2000. Geographic Area: Iowa. Vol. 2003. Washington, D.C.: U.S. Census Bureau.

———. 2004. Profile of General Demographic Characteristics 2000 (State of Iowa). Washington, D.C.: U.S. Census Bureau.

Van Wolputte, Steven. 2004. Hang on to your self: of bodies, embodiment, and selves. *Annual Review of Anthropology* 33: 251–269.

Verhaak, Peter F. M., Monique J.W.M. Heijmans, Loe Peters, and Micke Rijken. 2005. Chronic disease and mental disorder. *Social Science and Medicine* 60(4): 789–797.

Vernon, G. M. 1989. Parkinson's disease. *Journal of Neuroscience Nursing* 21(5): 273–284.

Victor, Daryl, and Cheryl Waters. 2003. Monoamine oxidase inhibitors in Parkinson's disease. In *Handbook of Parkinson's Disease*, ed. R. Pahwa, K. E. Lyons, and W. C. Koller. New York: Marcel Dekker.

Wallhagan, M. I., and M. Brod. 1997. Perceived control and well-being in Parkinson's disease. *Western Journal of Nursing Research* 19(1): 11–31.

Ware, John E. 1993. *SF-36 Health Survey Manual and Interpretation Guide*. Boston: Health Institute, New England Medical Center.

———. 1995. The status of health assessment 1994. *Annual Review of Public Health* 16: 327–354.

Ware, John E., and Cathy Donald Sherbourne. 1992. The MOS 36-Item Short Form Health Survey (SF-36). *Medical Care* 30(6): 473–481.

Wechsler, L. S., H. Checkoway, G. M. Franklin, and L. G. Costa. 1991. A pilot study of occupational and environmental risk factors for Parkinson's disease. *Neurotoxicology* 12: 387–392.

Whettan-Goldstein, K., F. A. Sloan, E. Kulas, T. M. Cutson, and M. Schenkman. 1997. The burdens of Parkinson's disease on society. *Journal of the American Geriatrics Society* 45: 844–849.

Whyte, Susan Reynolds, and Benedicte Ingstad. 1995. Disability and culture: an overview. In *Disability and Culture*, ed. B. Ingstad and S. R. Whyte. Berkeley: University of California Press.

Wielinski, C. L., C. E. Erikson-Davis, R. Wichmann, M. Walde-Douglas, and S. A. Parashos. 2005. Falls and injuries resulting from falls among patients with Parkinson's disease and other parkinsonian syndromes. *Movement Disorders* 20(4): 410–415.

Williams, Simon. 2000. Chronic illness as biographical disruption or biographical disruption as chronic illness? Reflections on a core concept. *Sociology of Health and Illness* 22(1): 40–67.

Wolf, Margery. 1992. *A Thrice-Told Tale: Feminism, Postmodernism, and Ethnographic Responsibility.* Stanford, Calif.: Stanford University Press.

Wood, B. H., J. A. Bilclough, A. Bowron, and R. W. Walker. 2002. Incidence and prediction of falls in Parkinson's disease: a prospective multidisciplinary study. *Journal of Neurology, Neurosurgery, and Psychiatry* 72(6): 721–725.

Wood, B. H., and R. W. Walker. 2005. Osteoporosis in Parkinson's disease. *Movement Disorders* 20(12): 1636–1640.

Woodruff-Pak, Diana S. 1997. *The Neuropsychology of Aging.* Malden, Mass.: Blackwell.

Youdim, M.B.H., and P. Riederer. 1997. Understanding Parkinson's disease. *Scientific American* 276(1): 52–59.

Young, Allan. 1982. The anthropologies of illness and sickness. *Annual Review of Anthropology* 11(1): 257–285.

Zimmerman, Sheryl, Philip D. Sloane, and J. Kevin Eckert. 2001. *Assisted Living: Needs, Practices, and Policies in Residential Care for the Elderly.* Baltimore: Johns Hopkins University Press.

INDEX

ABOUT THE AUTHOR

Samantha Solimeo is a lecturer in the Department of Sociology and Anthropology at North Carolina State University. She completed her graduate work in feminist anthropology in 2005 and in gerontological public health in 2003 at the University of Iowa. Subsequently she completed a postdoctoral fellowship in medical anthropology at the Duke University Center for the Study of Aging and Human Development. In addition to teaching courses on aging, human development, and cultural anthropology, Solimeo is an active member of the American Anthropological Association, the Gerontological Society of America, and the Association for Anthropology and Gerontology. Her research emphasizes the cultural construction of somatic experience at the intersection of chronic conditions, narrative, and identity. She is currently working on a study of masculinity, aging, and risk in the case of osteoporosis.

Printed in the United States
142482LV00001B/1/P